Susan's Song

The Endearing Story Of A Woman's Battle With Breast Cancer

By Susan & Gil Gerretsen

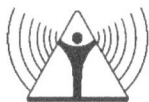

Published by BizTrek Books
A Division of BizTrek Inc.
Taylors, SC 29687
+1 (864) 268-5300

ISBN: 978-1-947190-05-4
Printed in the United States of America

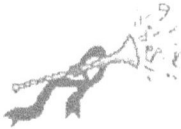

Friday, March 28, 2003

If God brings me to it, he will bring me through it

May there be peace within you today. May you trust God that you are exactly where you are meant to be. "I believe that friends are quiet angels who lift us to our feet when our wings have trouble remembering how to fly."

Hello Everyone

We received some frightening news yesterday. I have been diagnosed with breast cancer and will undergo bilateral mastectomies on Saturday morning, April 5. The cancer is in its early stages, and the surgeon is optimistic. I have also seen a plastic surgeon and will have reconstruction at the same time. The procedure itself should take 4-5 hours. I have had the privilege of choosing the surgeons, OR team and recovery room staff. I am very comfortable with the decision to have the surgery and with the people who will be caring for me during that time.

We want to ask for your prayers during this time. A friend sent the above e-mail to me yesterday, and it couldn't have come at a better time. It reminded me that there is a Higher Power and that whatever happens, it is in His hands. We have been so blessed with so many wonderful friendships over the years and appreciate all your support. Please remember us in your prayers next Saturday.

Thank you for being our friends.

Love,
Susan

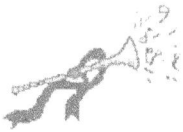

Wednesday, April 9, 2003

Hello Again

I wanted to thank you all for your prayers, calls, cards, flowers and gifts during the last few days. Saturday was rough, but I was able to go home from the hospital Sunday afternoon. I still cannot lift anything and am resting most of the time. I see both Dr. Bour and Dr. Graham on Friday and our earnest prayer now is for negative lymph nodes.

The pain is tolerable, and I'm walking around the house pretty well. I have progressed to washing my own hair and doing small things for myself. Every time I get achy and tired, I simply say, "I don't have breast cancer anymore," and then it all falls into perspective.

We really appreciate each of you and all your good thoughts, deeds and prayers. Please continue to pray that we are open to God's will in our lives and that whatever He brings to us, we will accept with grace and peace. Thank you for your friendship and for your continued support.

We love each of you.
Susan

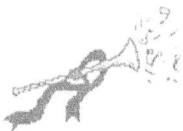

Saturday, April 12, 2003

Hello Everyone

It's hard to believe that just about one week ago now I was preparing to go to the hospital for my surgery. I've had a good week—am able to do most things for myself now. I still have lifting restrictions—yes, poor Gil is suffering the miseries of waiting on me, but doing so very graciously. I'm trying not to wear him out!!

We saw both surgeons yesterday and they were pleased with my progress. My plastic surgeon removed two of the four drains I have (which are probably my biggest complaint!) and we hope to get the other two removed late next week. I'm sore and tender, but able to walk and plan to enjoy our beautiful weather and be outside as much as possible in the coming weeks.

All of the breast tissue that was removed was negative for cancer, and I am still glad I made the decision I did to have a bilateral mastectomy. The bad news is that of 11 lymph nodes that were removed from my right side, four had cancer in them. It's very small in each node, but I didn't get a clean bill of health. This means I will have an appointment with an oncologist next week to begin chemotherapy. (My surgeon did say the type of breast cancer I have is estrogen receptor positive, which means it will be very responsive to the chemo.) Of course, we were disappointed with this news and I don't look forward to the treatments, but we still believe God has a reason for everything, so we are trying to be thankful for the lessons we are to learn. I'm not able to thank God yet for this, but at least I can be honest with Him when I tell Him I'm trying to be grateful, but it's hard!!

We have very much appreciated all your wonderful support—e-mails, cards, flowers, food, gifts, calls and so many other ways you have surrounded us with you love and care. Please continue to pray for us that we will be strong and know that you are in our prayers as well. God has blessed us with us with so much—both tangible and intangible and we are so grateful for your prayers and concern.

Love,
Susan

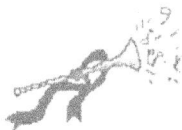

Thursday, April 24, 2003

The good news I am beginning to have shape in my chest again!!! I saw my plastic surgeon on Monday and FINALLY got the remaining two drains pulled—I don't think anything has ever felt so good. After the initial stinging, it felt sooooo good to be free and be able to move without worrying about bumping or pulling the drains. I walked three miles on Tuesday and Wednesday and really enjoyed swinging my arms and the freedom of movement I have now. I also can drive, although not very comfortably with a stick shift, but I do have my wheels back!!! If you see me coming towards you on the road, you may want to be extra cautious!! I am pretty much independent now—I can even take a shower all by myself!! My doctor also began filling my tissue expanders and I now have boob-lets. They aren't very big, but they are present and I have graduated to wearing a bra again. In the right clothes, no one can even tell I've had surgery and I'm very excited to "see what develops" in the next month or so.

As you may know, I had my initial oncologist visit yesterday. Gil and I both LOVED Dr. Giguere. What a compassionate, patient and kind man God has provided to care for us. He has been doing oncology for 20 years, with the majority of that time specializing in breast cancer treatment. He spent about an hour with us yesterday, explaining things, outlining our choices, answering questions and going over what to expect. In such a frightening situation, it helps to know someone this wonderful is my "team leader." We both felt very pleased and comfortable that he will be overseeing my treatment this year.

I had blood drawn yesterday and I understand this will be a weekly occurrence from now on. I also have to have a bone scan on Tuesday. And sometime in the next week, I will have to make one more trip to the OR to have a life port placed in my upper chest. This will be the access to my venous system and it means I won't have to be stuck every time I have an infusion or lab work is needed. So it's a good thing, since they were digging in my arm for about 10 minutes yesterday for blood!!

I will begin chemo soon—probably the second week of May. I will be given two drugs concurrently three weeks apart, four times. Then they will switch to another drug and give that every three weeks, four times. So the chemo regimen lasts 24 weeks. I will lose my hair (but who wants to shave their legs in the summer anyway??), and Dr. Giguere said my treatment was aggressive because my tumor was aggressive and with positive lymph nodes, and because I was so young (now do you see why I loved him?), he really wanted to impact any possible residual tumor. After the chemo is completed, I will have six weeks of radiation therapy to my chest wall. Apparently this is like the old Raid commercial that said it "kills bugs dead." If there is any cancer left in my body, it will be killed dead.

Dr. Giguere participates in research (mostly with Duke University) and offered us options regarding anti-hormone therapies and several other trials I may elect to participate in, including strengthening (diet and exercise). He has also asked the pathologist to send my biopsy out for additional testing at the DNA level, so if there is something genetic, there is another treatment modality to deal with this. So this will be year of learning for both of us. However, by Christmas it will all be over and our new life can begin. My 42nd year will not be my best year, but we are looking forward to the future and what it holds for us.

It was a day of very mixed emotions. When I was walking across the parking lot to enter the Cancer Center, I got teary because the last time I was there was to take my mother two summers ago. I was somewhat familiar with the staff and the procedures, but it's always different when you are the patient. Everyone we encountered yesterday was very nice and caring and I hear it just gets better as the staff gets to know you and your family throughout treatment. This is still fresh and we have to assimilate a lot of information in a short period of time. And if you don't know already, I am a very high control person, so part of my fear is that I have lost control over my own body.

We did have some humor in the lobby yesterday. If you don't remember, my husband has alopecia and hasn't had any hair for nearly 20 years. As I was watching people come and go, I was sniffling and scared. One gentleman (who obviously shaved what little hair he had left) came up to Gil and asked how he got his head so smooth. I had to laugh at myself because as I was sitting there frightened and intimidated, I realized everyone thought poor Gil was the patient, not me!!! Gil explained to the man that his head looked like that "naturally" and the man told him how good he looked and that he only needed an earring to be perfect!! Now for those of you who know Gil, you can imagine his reaction to being told he needed an earring!!! Then the man said he got his hairdo from brain tumors. Whoa!! How's that for some perspective???

Once again, we have to thank you for all your prayers and support. As we go through this "ordeal" we are so grateful to all of you for the cards, e-mails, prayers and other kindnesses you have shown us. It's not going to be easy, but when we look back on this, I plan to have laughter to go with the tears. Thank you for all your caring!!

Love,
Susan

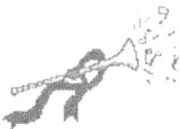

Sunday, May 4, 2003

Good Morning Everyone

It's 46 degrees here this morning after a stormy evening yesterday. Before I drag Gil out of bed for our walk, I thought I'd take a few minutes to let you know how we're doing and what's happened this past week. It's been a very busy, productive week and we've learned a lot.

Monday I saw my plastic surgeon and got my boob-lets enlarged some more. Every week he fills the tissue expanders with saline, until I tell him I can't breathe. This week I managed 70 cc in one side and 80 cc in the other. It's not fun being stuck with needles in an already tender chest area, but the results are worth the pain. Soon, I'll be writing to you about my boobies.

Tuesday I had a bone scan at my hospital. I had to be there at 10:45 for yet another IV injection, then "go away" until 2:00 for the actual scan. I saw a lot of friends from Surgery (everyone wanted to hug me, but with my newly enlarged chest, that wasn't possible) and got taken to lunch by my bosses. I did learn I will have a position with the hospital when this is all over and I'm ready to return to work (sometime next year). It was GREAT to see the wonderful group of folks I work with and share some tears and laughter with them. The best news of that day is that my bone scan is negative, which means the cancer has not spread. I learned that the type of breast cancer I have loves to migrate to the bones, and mine was caught early enough that this has not happened!! Several times at the oncologist on Thursday, I heard the phrase "non-metastatic disease" and it was wonderful. Actually, I have the second-best cancer (is that an oxymoron or what??!!) a person can have.

Wednesday I went to my old hospital and had a life port installed in my upper left chest wall. It was minor outpatient surgery and I'm thankful to have the port. As someone who has dental floss for veins, this means I don't have to be stuck every time someone needs to administer medication or to draw blood for lab work (which will happen on an at least weekly basis over the next year). The spot is still tender, but I'm very thankful the port is in place. Once again I saw lots of friends and received lots of hugs, presents (I LOVE presents) and words of comfort and support. I'm really thankful to work with such a great group of people. A good friend took me to lunch and then we meandered our way home—stopping at another friend's to see their new baby horse and just visit. It was a very positive afternoon, and I slept really well Wednesday night.

Thursday we went back to the oncologist for a three-hour visit!! We learned that my cancer was very positive for a specific oncogene (cancer-causing gene) and that I am eligible for an additional study and drug that work at the genetic level. The study is sponsored by Duke University and my oncologist is one of the leading researchers in this study. So after receiving the first round of chemo for 12 weeks, there could be a drug that is given in conjunction with the second round of chemo (and this second drug is given every week for a year) that will help with the genetic expression of the tumor. It's fascinating to learn; I just wish I wasn't the guinea pig!! But again, I am thankful for the additional drugs that we have to help win this war.

I met three wonderful nurses at the Cancer Center, and they were very patient and answered my zillion questions. I was even brave enough to go see the area where chemotherapy is administered and meet some of that staff as well. For me, knowledge and information instill power in me over this situation. I am trying to take baby steps in this process, so that when I actually begin the chemo in a couple of weeks, I'll feel empowered and as ready as I can be. I also learned that my infusions will probably take no more than four hours, and then I'll be done. I asked to start May 13, and to have my chemo on Tuesdays.

This week, I have two doctor appointments on Monday (yes, my boob-lets will be even larger by Monday evening). On Tuesday, I need to have lots of "pre-protocol" (notice how we're stepping around the word chemotherapy) blood work drawn (thank God for life ports). Then it's back to the hospital for "pre-protocol" chest X-ray, EKG and MUGA scan—which is a test that looks at your heart. Apparently, one of the chemotherapeutic agents is very stressful to the heart, and they want baseline values for all these tests before we "dive in."

Then I'm taking the rest of the week off to rest and prepare for the following week. Gil's birthday is Thursday and we've decided to be people and enjoy ourselves, instead of being patients and worrying about cancer. We are so thankful for all your cards, e-mails, phone calls and all the ways you demonstrate support and love to us. God has surrounded us with such a great group of friends and we feel like we have an army right beside us as we march through this battle. Thank you for being GREAT friends!!

Love,
Susan

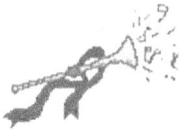

Sunday, May 11, 2003

Hello Everyone

This has been another week of learning for us. We continue to be blessed in so many ways by all of you and we are so grateful for each of you!!

Monday I had my weekly visit with my plastic surgeon—and I think we have graduated from boob-lets to boobs now. I had no idea my muscles could be re-configured in this way, but I am developing quite a bust line!! I am so very thankful for this particular doctor and his gift that he so willingly shares with me. We will continue to fill the expanders and re-shape my chest for a while longer. Then that process will be "on hold" until next year, after all the other treatments are completed. We saw friends on Friday night that were quite impressed with what has been accomplished in four weeks!!

Tuesday I had to go to the Cancer Center for "pre-treatment" lab work. The nurse accessed my life port and withdrew seven tubes of blood from it!! I was so thankful for that port, because I can't imagine how many times I would have been stuck in the arm otherwise!! I also met Dr. Giguere's chemotherapy nurse and was further oriented to what will happen on Tuesday. I felt very brave going into the Cancer Center all by myself, considering two weeks ago I couldn't even walk across the parking lot without crying!! One of the two research nurses that I have "clicked" with also sat down with me and went over the scans and tests I have had done previously. She told me she wanted me to understand that I don't have cancer—surgically, it was removed from my body before it had any chance to spread. The reason I am having chemotherapy is so it won't come back, in case there is one cell hiding out somewhere, waiting to grow. Then chemo is a systemic treatment that will reach every cell in my body and if one of them has the ability to become cancerous, it will be killed. This really helped my perspective and attitude towards the chemo. There are so many people that aren't as healthy as me and I was forced to acknowledge that I was indeed fortunate that my disease was caught early and is treatable.

After leaving the Cancer Center, I went to the hospital for a series of "pre-treatment" tests (again!!). Note how everyone is avoiding the work "chemo" and instead saying "treatment." The first test was a MUGA scan, which looks at the heart. Adriamycin (one of the first chemo agents I will receive) is very taxing on the heart, and we need to have baseline values before I receive any "treatment". They had to start an IV in my hand and withdraw 5 cc of blood. That blood undergoes several processes, but eventually it tagged radioactively and re-injected into your body. Then you are positioned under the scanner and have to sit still for 20 minutes.

The good news is that my heart is in good shape—I guess it's all the walking I've done lately. The next test was just a chest X-ray and mine was perfect. Then I had to go for an EKG—again it was perfect, so even though it was an exhausting afternoon, the results were worth the effort. I came home and slept for almost 14 hours straight!!

Wednesday afternoon I got a call from the nurse at the Cancer Center and she told me all my tests were normal. Of course they haven't done a head CT, so I'm not sure about that diagnosis :-)!! She answered another round of questions from me and I feel ready to start this process on Tuesday.

Thursday and Friday I spent cleaning the house at my own pace. Gil's birthday was Thursday and we had dinner in town that night. On Friday we had a cookout and had friends over. It was a great evening of fun, food and fellowship. Poor Gil has been in the background so much lately, and it was a great night for him. We had lots of help with preparations, cooking and cleanup, so it wasn't too much work for any of us. Plus we have a fridge full of great leftovers!!

On Friday I walked 5 miles and on Saturday we both walked 6 miles. It has been very warm and muggy here lately, so you really work up a sweat. When we got home yesterday, we decided we were already "dirty," so we both worked outside for hours. Gil came in at dark!! Today our big plans are to get our summer garden plants in the ground and read the Sunday paper. I think we'll be able to accomplish that!!

Tomorrow I am getting my hair cut off. I have been growing it out for an organization called "Locks of Love," which makes wigs for children without hair (due to chemo, etc.). I had planned to grow it to my waist, and then cut it off at my shoulders, but you know what they say about life happening when you've made other plans!! It is halfway down my back and we think if we cut if off about 2 inches long all over, I'll have enough to donate. So at least that will be a positive thing to come out of this!! I also see my plastic surgeon again tomorrow, and yes, I will be a "bigger" person for the experience!!

Tuesday I will start chemotherapy. Gil is taking the day off to go with me. There have been so many advances in the drugs in recent years that I am trying to keep an open mind about all of it. I will lose my hair, but as far as the nausea and other horror stories we have all heard, the nurses at the Cancer Center tell me that everyone is different and that I may not even get sick!! They said I will probably feel flu-like on Tuesday night, and then feel tired Wednesday, Thursday and Friday. By the weekend, I should be back to

11

normal. This will go on for seven more cycles, every three weeks. So I've decided the way to get through it is to see that for every four crummy days I have, I'll have 17 good days!! I am excited that the chemo will completely eradicate any lingering "bad" cells from my body, and I'm grateful for the offers from friends to go with me. And after Tuesday, I'll only have 7 more treatments!!

Please keep us in your prayers as we face this challenging week. We both know there is a reason for everything and that ultimately there is a much Higher Power than us. We appreciate each of you and all the ways you uplift us!! Have a GREAT week!!

Love,
Susan

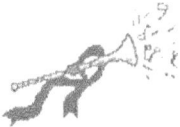

Tuesday, May 20, 2003

Hello Again

I think I've finally re-surfaced after last week!! Thank you for all you inquiries-I have been overwhelmed recuperating from the effects of chemo. However, now we know what to expect and will be better prepared next time.

Monday was most traumatic for me. Probably the most ironic thing about this whole ordeal is that I was growing my hair out to cut off and give away to Locks of Love. For those of you who don't know what that is, it's an organization that makes wigs for children with alopecia who otherwise couldn't afford to have hair. This process has been a year and a half in the making, and the plan was to grow my hair to my waist, then cut it off at my shoulders. Well, life certainly had other plans for me. I went Monday and had my beautiful mid-back locks shorn-yes, like a lamb to the slaughter!! My hair has not been this short in 30 years, but I keep reminding myself that in another week I would be grateful for at least this much hair. I cried for weeks preceding this event and it was very emotionally painful for me. However, there is always a silver lining, and mine is that I was able to donate a 14 inch long, 2 inch diameter ponytail to some child who needs it more than me. And my hair will grow back!! I still have my hair today-the folks at the Cancer Center tell me to expect it to fall out in 10-14 days from the initial chemo treatment, and we are on day 8. I have chosen not to wear a wig-we will probably also donate the money I would have spent on that to Locks of Love. Besides, it's summer and hot (well, it's supposed to be here, but it isn't!) and the best news is I won't have to shave my legs all summer!!

Tuesday was the BIG day for us. Gil took the day off and took me to my first chemo treatment. I have been walking religiously since surgery and the exciting news when I stepped on the scale at the Cancer Center was I had lost 6 ½ pounds!! That was a GREAT start to the day!! We arrived at 10:45 and with all the teaching they do and preparation, it was about 12:30 when they finally accessed my life port and started the IV-and I'll say it again, thank God for life ports!! The nurse first gave me a new anti-nausea medicine that was developed specifically for chemo patients called Anzemet (a miracle drug, to say the least!) with a steroid called Decadron (that actually gives the Anzemet a boost to work even better). I got some IV fluid, then the nurse came in with Adriamycin (the first chemotherapeutic agent), about 1:15. It looks like red Kool-Aid and they give it over about 5 minutes by pushing it through the IV. In order to decrease the mouth sores that Adriamycin can cause, they also have you suck on Popsicles while they are giving it, so your mouth and gums are cold and the blood vessels are constricted. This way, the medicine doesn't get to those tissues quite as easily!! Then they ran some more IV fluid, and hung the bag of Cytoxan (the second agent), which ran in over an hour. They want you to eat and drink throughout the process (we actually brought a cooler with fruit and cheese and drinks in it) and I couldn't believe I was able to eat while receiving chemo, but I did!! We were out of there by 3:00 and even had prescriptions filled, went to the bank and grocery store on the way home!! I continued to eat Tuesday evening and was fine.

The next five days I'm calling "the good, the bad, the ugly, the bad and the good." Wednesday I was bloated and gassy, but not nauseated!! They had given me oral Anzemet to take for the three days following chemotherapy. I ate healthy and even exercised (yes, the day after chemo!!). Thursday became the bad-I wasn't quite nauseated, but felt like I was going to be any minute. I continued to eat lightly and sparingly, but mostly laid around and did very little all day. Friday was ugly-nausea all day. I had two pieces of dry toast the whole day and by Friday night I was in the bathroom-I'll spare you the gory details. Saturday was back to bad-I wasn't really nauseated but felt "yucky" and didn't eat all day. During "the bad and ugly" days, food was completely revolting to me-I had to turn off commercials on TV, I couldn't stand a lot of odors, and motion (like the dog wagging his tail) even upset me!! Then we got back to "the good." Sunday morning I slept till 10:00 and woke up wanting hot chocolate and plain pancakes!! My long-suffering husband was excited to be able to fix something and have me eat it. He even took me for a drive Sunday evening-we had to go to the grocery store (a most exciting adventure!) and it was GREAT to get out of the house.

Yesterday I felt good enough to walk, however it took me an hour to walk two miles. One of the effects of chemo is that it destroys good cells along with the bad, so I am probably a little anemic. But I did walk, and then slept for three hours!! I also cooked supper for the first time in a week. And I am making spaghetti sauce even as I type-so I am better. I will also have low white blood cell counts and have been told to stay home this week except for doctor appointments ... and to stay away from other people as much as possible. Next week is supposed to be the "fun" week in all this, and then we repeat the process again, starting June 3. But we have the initial treatment done, and there are only seven to go. I have to remember that the second part of chemo is therapy and that means it's doing good things. If I only have three really bad days per 21 days, I can't complain. And to see some of the folks in the Cancer Center who are also patients, I am VERY THANKFUL for my diagnosis and treatment.

I'm also thankful for a very loving and supportive husband and for each of you. At times like these, you really do reflect upon all your blessings. I do have so very much to be grateful for, and I can say that God has been very good to me. Hope you have a great week!!

Love,
Susan

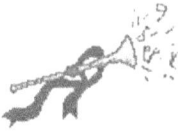

Tuesday, May 27, 2003

Hello Everyone

Hope you had a great holiday weekend. We were able to get our five acres mowed—I spent about five hours on the riding mower and amazed even myself!! I have decided that if I ever give up nursing as a career, my new job will be as the Zamboni driver at the ice rink!! We had dinner "in town" with friends on Saturday night, then Sunday was literally a day of rest for me!!
Monday we met friends for breakfast "in town", then went shopping for Gil's belated birthday present. He had decided he wanted a digital camera, but that's not something I'm comfortable selecting him, so we shopped together. He didn't find what he wanted at the stores, but was able to go on-line and get the exact camera he had chosen. After that four-hour trip around town, I came home and took a wonderful three-hour nap!! I just love naps and it was very refreshing.

We both walked all three weekend days and it felt soooo good. Remember last Monday, when I could barely struggle two miles and it took me an hour? Well I'm seeing lots of progress. Today I walked to our neighbors' driveway—two and a half miles each way and did it in an hour and 15 minutes!! Their street address is Landrum, and it tickles me to say I've walked to another city! I'm pretty tired and don't know if I'll amount to much the rest of the day, but it's certainly an improvement over last week. My goal is to be able to make it to the end of our road (which is three miles each way) before each of my next chemo treatments. I've already told Gil we'll be going that far this coming weekend. I somehow manage to wake up in a pretzel shape each morning, which makes me stiff and sore (or as they say around here, "all stove up"). If I walk first thing, then take a blistering hot shower, I can usually get by with Tylenol, or even nothing. I have decided that there is nothing bad about walking, and it's such a positive thing to do for myself.

I saw the nurse practitioner at Dr. Giguere's office on Friday. My counts had dropped significantly, which means the chemo is working inside my body. I had also lost 11 pounds since the previous Tuesday. I was thrilled, but they were not!! I told her about my experience on the weekend with the nausea and anorexia, and they have switched my anti-nausea medicine. The new drug is called Emend and it's just been approved by the FDA in the past month. I have samples to take next week and am hopeful I will have a better experience next time. If not, it's 21 bad days left, and what's 21 days in my whole lifetime? Very do-able, I say, especially since I will be assured I'm not going to have breast cancer ever again!!

I also saw my plastic surgeon on Friday. Once again, I am pleased at our progress and excited about what's to come. There is very definitely a bust line present now, and each time I go to his office, there is improvement. This is not an episode, but a journey, and it takes time for him to create something out of nothing. I'm very thankful to have such a compassionate and caring person helping me, not to mention that he's a very gifted surgeon.

And now, about my hair. It is still with us. They told me to expect the "shedding" to occur 10-14 days after chemo, and today is day 14. I feel like I'm "living on borrowed time" in some ways, but am thankful I still have it. Gil took me to the wig shop last Friday and I ended up getting a wig after all.

It was much less expensive that I had thought. We showed the lady my driver's license picture and told her we wanted to see something similar to that. The first wig she put on my head had tears popping into my eyes, because I looked like me again. If you know I've had chemo, you'll know I'm wearing a wig, but if the general population sees me, it isn't obvious at all. I also got a "fringe" that fits just around the outside of my head (kind of like Friar Tuck) that goes with my hats. Now it's really difficult to tell anything when I wear a hat. So I feel much better about the hair issue.

I do have a funny story to tell you. On Friday when I was in the lobby at the Cancer Center, several of the nurses were stopping to tell me how much they liked my hair. I was trying to be gracious and say thank you. There was a beautiful woman sitting across from me with a gorgeous scarf under her hat. We went to our separate appointments, and happened to be leaving together. In the parking lot, I stopped her and asked her where she had gotten her scarf. She told me it was a gift from a friend, and then congratulated me on my hair growing back. She told me it was beautiful and asked if I was excited.

Once again, I was humbled to realize how self-involved I had been. I told her my hair had not come out yet and how upset I had been at cutting 14 inches off of it. We ended up talking for about 20 minutes and she is a very sick lady. She has lymphoma and was on her way to get a platelet transfusion. Yet she still had a beautiful smile on her face and told me she would say a prayer for me!! Wow!! It's amazing how God continues to work on me in this situation. I am so fortunate in so many ways, and He is really good at pointing those out to me. He's using humor (which I respond to very well) to make me see things in a new perspective, then be able to laugh at myself and not be so serious all the time. I am grateful for this time to work on myself—physically, emotionally and spiritually.

This is my "off week" which I'm told is the week everyone looks forward to. I still have lingering fatigue, but it's nothing like last week. I just have to rest between activities, but that's not a problem. I'm simply going to enjoy each day and be thankful for all the blessings that come my way. I hope this week will be the start of a great summer for you!! Have a great week!!

Love,
Susan

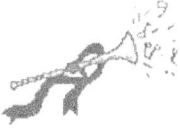

Monday, June 2, 2003

Hello Everyone,

It's a gorgeous afternoon-our thermometer says 78 degrees, sunny and breezy. And I am inside, purposely not working on my suntan!! We have hummingbirds fighting over our feeders and our first calla lilies are open. I got about half of our summer bedding plants put into the ground last night, and when it cools down a little more, I hope to get the rest put in tonight. There is so much for which we have to be thankful!!

This past week was hard in one aspect and GREAT in others. My hair finally started coming out on Wednesday and it is almost completely gone. I have probably lost 80 to 85 percent from my poor head. I wore a hat "out" for the first time Saturday evening, and was very self-conscious. Today I wore my "fringe with a big pink hat and got a lot of compliments. So this is just something I have to get over!! It's going to take a little time. I am still startled when I look in the mirror. And my scalp is very tender, but itchy!! However, the biggest disappointment is that I still have to shave my legs!! Can someone please tell me where the justice in this is???

I have been selected to participate in a research study through Duke University for "young patients with breast cancer." My study focuses on diet and exercise for the six months I will be receiving chemotherapy. I received a large box in the mail Wednesday and it contains a walkman, an exercise ball, stretchy bands, a heart monitor, video and audio tapes and all kinds of other goodies. I wore an activity monitor Thursday, Friday and Saturday-it's about the size of a pager, and I mailed it and lots of survey information back to the research coordinator at Duke this morning. I will wear this monitor again in three months and at the end of the study. (I was able to walk 37 miles last week-a new record for me!! I am eager to step on the scale at the doctor's office on Wednesday.) My diet is high calcium, moderate fat, moderate protein and high fruits and vegetables. Thank goodness this is summertime-when the fresh fruit and veggies are plentiful!! The purpose of all this is to evaluate how my specific chemo regimen affects my health. About two weeks ago, I had a bone scan and a body mass index done, and will have another at the end of the study. The goal is to help me manage weight-the average "young" breast cancer patient gains 22 lbs. during chemo, or has a significant loss of lean muscle mass and gain of fatty tissue due to inactivity and fatigue. Also, the chemo I'm receiving "attacks" bone and we want to maintain as much healthy bone as possible, while eradicating any remaining cancer cells. I'm excited about this opportunity and looking forward to what we'll see in October.

I saw my orthodontist this morning-since I won't see him again until July 14, I now have red, white and blue rings on my braces!! It gives me something else to look at when I see myself in the mirror. I also saw my plastic surgeon today-I am quite pleased with our results, even though I am not able to breathe deeply just now!! Oh well-as the adage goes, no pain, no gain. And we are definitely seeing "gain!!"

This week will bring challenges to us-please keep us in your prayers and thoughts on Wednesday. I have my next round of chemo starting at about 11:30. I was supposed to go tomorrow, but Dr. Giguere is not in the office, and I have to see him before I receive any treatments. (I'm sure he was completely unaware it was ME who wanted to come on Tuesday when his scheduling conflict occurred!!!) I start taking my new medication on Wednesday morning and am hopeful that it will work better than last time. If not, by this time next week, I'll have three more yucky days behind me and will only have 18 left!! We'll let you know next week!! My good friend Janet is meeting me at the Cancer Center on Wednesday, so I'll have a chemo buddy with me. This is just too hard for me to do alone-and poor Gil can't always take a day off to spend with me. Most people have an "entourage" with them and it's comforting to have a familiar, friendly face sitting right next to you when they start infusing the drugs.

I hope you have a great week!!

Love,
Susan

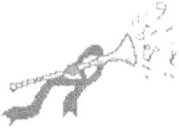

Wednesday, June 11, 2003

Good Morning!!!

We have just finished a very challenging week, but we were able to find a blessing each day. Let me start by thanking each of you for your prayers, calls, cards, e-mail, gifts and all the other ways you continue to support us. We have been overwhelmed by the kindness of our family and friends and we are so thankful for each of you.

Remember I was trying a new anti-nausea medicine when I had chemo this time? Well, we discovered Emend doesn't work for me!! I have to say that chemo knocked me on my rear end and kicked me in the guts this time. I had my chemo last Wednesday and was nauseated as soon as I got home (about 45 minutes after it was finished infusing). I continued to be very sick and called the cancer center Friday to see what else I could take. They gave me oral Zofran (which we use in surgery for anti-nausea) and it helped. Some. I couldn't eat at all on Friday or Saturday. Sunday morning I started feeling a little better and was able to eat dry toast, but was in the bathroom again by Sunday night. Monday afternoon I began to feel like I was crawling from the pit, and by yesterday evening I felt better. I see the nurse practitioner this Friday (the 13th) and will have a big discussion with her about what we're going to do differently next time. I had heard that chemo could be cumulative and that each time gets progressively worse. I choose not to believe this, but instead to think we are faced with a challenge and have to keep trying different options until we find what does work. If I have to, I'll go back to what I took the first time and have three bad days instead of five!!

Poor Gil was also very challenged with keeping smells, sounds, pictures, motion, etc. to a bare minimum. At one point, I was sitting in a chair, and holding onto the bookcase beside it because the room was spinning so badly!! He has been such a patient and supportive person—it can't be easy living like this for almost a week at a time. He even ate in the kitchen under the exhaust fan so I wouldn't smell his food!! I'm very thankful for a kind and patient man!!

The other issue I had trouble with this time was the taste in my mouth. Last time everything tasted metallic. Chemo indiscriminately kills all rapidly-dividing cells in the body and your gastrointestinal tract is lined with just such cells. So from day 2 to about day 6, I had a vile taste in my mouth. I tried mouthwash, tooth brushing every hour or so, chewing gum (with my orthodontist's blessing) and everything else I could think of, but nothing helped. I have to drink at least 6 glasses of water daily to not become dehydrated (which will also contribute to the nausea) and for two days, even that made me gag!!! So today, I relished my cereal and milk and am thankful food tastes good again!!!

Despite being sick on Saturday, I was able to begin the exercise program I am participating in with Duke. I am calling these my Dookey Exercises!! (I have decided those giant balls are nothing more than torture devices!!) Seriously, I have strengthening and stretching exercises for the lower body and they do make me sweat!! I am supposed to do these every other day, and then do some form of aerobic exercise on the "off" days. I never knew you were supposed to have muscles on your legs—mine are so well protected under all that fat!! I am sore in places I didn't know I had!! I did walk a mile in 45 minutes yesterday—and will hopefully continue to improve on this until I have once again conquered cardiac hill before my next session.

Our week also brought great beauty. Probably the most touching moment was last Wednesday when I went for chemo. Remember me telling you about the sick lady with the beautiful scarf that I talked to in the parking lot the previous visit? When I arrived, one of the nurses had a gift bag for me and said she had been asked by a patient to give it to me. When I opened it up, inside was the same scarf and the sweetest note from the patient, telling me she remembered how upset I was about my hair, and that she wanted me to have the scarf and know that she was praying for me. Once again, I was humbled by the kindness of someone I hardly know, who, despite being very sick herself, was reaching out to me. I think God continues to place just such people in my path to remind me of His presence throughout this time.

Speaking of my hair, I think I look like Linus in the Peanuts comic strip— little strings of wispy hair that are thinning each day. However, I am still having to shave my legs, and am ready for that to be over!! If you're going to mess with my hair, then you need to take ALL of it!!

Last night, we were in our garden for a few minutes. All of our seeds have sprouted and the tomatoes are blooming. Gil even has one baby pepper growing!! We looked over towards the chicken pen, and there was a deer in the yard. Well, it turn out she is very tame and Gil was able to pet her and get her to eat Saltine crackers from his hand. We often joke about living in "the sticks," but where else could you find something so charming in your own back yard? I did threaten him with torture if the "pet deer" gets into the garden!! We also have lots of hummingbirds fighting over the feeders and have bluebirds nesting again in the box outside our kitchen window. We did sit and watch lightning bugs last night for a few minutes. Even though this is my least favorite time of year because of the heat and humidity, I do love certain things about summer!!

Thank you again for all your love and support. May you be blessed this week, as we have been by you.

Love,
Susan

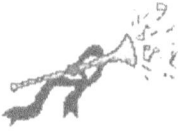

Monday, June 16, 2003

Hello Everyone

Hope your week is off to a great start. Ours is much better than last week, and we're thankful for that!!

I saw the nurse practitioner on Friday and she was dismayed to hear how sick I had been the previous week. I also had lost 8 pounds and for the first time in my life, someone told me I had lost too much weight!! (I was sure as long as I lived, I would never hear those words in reference to me, so I was quite surprised and delighted!!) So we spent about 30 minutes talking strategy for next week. The plan is for me to have the original drugs (Anzemet and Decadron) on Wednesday in the IV just before they infuse the chemo. Then I am to return to the cancer Thursday morning and again on Friday morning at 9:00 for additional anti-nausea medicine, steroids and fluids via IV. They will leave the access to my port in place so I don't have to get stuck each day and just "plug me in." We both felt I was becoming dehydrated and that was probably contributing to the nausea. This way, if I feel crummy, I don't have to worry about forcing nasty-tasting water down my throat. This combination worked well for me when I had my first chemo on Tuesday. I wasn't sick until Friday, so we both think the IV drugs will do well for me, and by Saturday, I should be "over the hump!" I'll take the oral Anzemet and Decadron on Saturday and Sunday. By Monday, I should be starting to rebound and hopefully feeling better. So once again, I am hopeful this will work.

My cell counts were down, of course, but not as bad as I had thought they would be. I was prepared to get a shot of Procrit, but I wasn't that depressed!! Yeah—the less needles the better. The nurse practitioner (who is also named Susan) was impressed as well. I asked her if all the exercising I'm doing is helping my counts not drop so significantly and she said I just had great bone marrow. So I asked her if I could quit exercising :-) and she said, NO!!! Oh well, you can't blame a girl for trying with all this heat and humidity!!

I also saw my plastic surgeon on Friday. That was another opportunity for four needles that I avoided. So Friday the 13th turned out to be a GREAT day for me!! We actually decided my tissue had not expanded enough to warrant filling the expanders more. I tease him that he has to be cruel to be kind, but this time he was very nice and didn't stick me at all!! We are now deciding how much "bigger" I need/want to be. And any of the men who read this, I am not taking a survey, but thank you anyway for your opinions!!! I may be almost "at capacity" on the non-cancer side and not too far away on the cancer side. Once I am at capacity, I won't have anything done until next year, when I am healed from radiation and am ready to have the expanders swapped for real implants.

This weekend was productive for us. We worked in the yard Saturday—actually Gil worked in the yard while I practiced my Zamboni skills on the riding mower. We were chased inside about 4:00 by a thunderstorm. Sunday I spent a lot of time resting and reading—my kind of day!! We both walked on Saturday morning—yes, I have once again conquered cardiac hill. And Sunday I did my Duke torture exercises!! I still can't believe there is that much muscle tissue on my legs for them to be so sore!! :-)

24

We were invited to a good friend's house to swim and it was wonderful. This pool is very secluded and private and we really had a nice time. I have to stay out of the sun this summer, so we swam in the evening. I hope we get to do that a lot more—it was really nice to cool off and feel so comfortable!!

While we were there, Gil and our friend were talking about how emotional I was last week. For some reason, hormonal or otherwise, I was very weepy and sad Monday and Tuesday. Gil said it was like living with the seven PMS dwarfs!! He specifically mentioned Sleepy, Weepy, Grumpy, and Pukey. I wonder who the other three dwarfs are??? Hmmm . . . I'm glad to see he hasn't lost his sense of humor in this challenging situation!!!

Well, that's about it for us. This is my "stay-at-home and be good" week since I'm immuno-suppressed. I have often joked that I would like to have the opportunity to become bored. I don't see that happening. I am dealing with residual fatigue and trying to once again get as strong as I can before my next treatment. Thank you again for your prayers and good thoughts—we are so appreciative of all your support!! Hope you have a great week!!

Love,
Susan

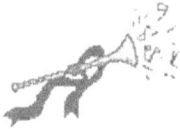

Tuesday, June 24, 2003

Hello again, Everyone!!

We both want to thank you for all your wonderful care this past week. We've received phone calls, e-mails, food, cards, visits and many other expressions of love and support. You are really helping us get through this "bump" in our road and we appreciate all you are doing for us—both things we know about, and the "behind the scenes" ways you are showing you care!!

It's been a good week for us. If you don't live in South Carolina, you should have visited this past weekend. We had "Chamber of Commerce" weather—low humidity, blue skies, high 70 degree temperatures—an absolutely perfect weekend!! We did our six-mile walk on Saturday morning and spent most of the rest of the day outside. Sunday was a rest day from all the activity on Saturday and we really enjoyed relaxing and reading. We had the windows open all weekend and our house smells fresh!!

We were able to enjoy dinner out four different times in the past week—it was great to visit with friends and get out of the house. (I'll bet I don't get fussed at tomorrow for losing too much weight this past week!!! :-)) We are both trying to make the best of our "good days" and not let chemo and cancer take over our lives. Even if we have 6 bad days, that leaves us 15 good days to get out and enjoy life!!! I still tire easily, so I have to pace myself—and that's hard. When you feel so good after feeling so bad, you just want to dive into every activity!!

My next dose of chemo is tomorrow, we are again asking for your prayers. I have been dreading it since the weekend, but I'm really trying to work on my attitude. This will be my third dose of four of the first drugs and that means I'll be 75% complete with Part 1. My friend Roxie is going with me this time—it's so nice to have "chemo buddies" and to be able to give Gil a break. We are trying another plan to deal with nausea and the other effects. I remain hopeful that we will find something that works for me!! I will be back at the Cancer Center on Thursday and Friday for IV fluids, anti-nausea medicine and steroids. Hopefully, this will get me through the roughest part, and this weekend will be better than the last.

I have a list of questions and comments for Dr. Giguere—the first issue is the fact that I still have to shave my legs!!! My head is almost completely bare—it just doesn't seem right that I should have such nice, thick hair on my legs!!!

I'm sure Dr. Giguere won't see this as a priority, but I do!!! :-)

Our 23rd wedding anniversary is Friday. I have often joked through the years that Gil is very fortunate and I am very patient to have lasted this long!!! I think this year that he gets the Medal of Honor to go with the "booby prize" (pun intended) he has for a wife right now!! We had our
anniversary dinner at home tonight, and will go out for a restaurant dinner in July. I'm so thankful to have someone who is going to tough this out with me and who I can depend on for everything—big, small, seemingly insignificant, gross, etc. It's wonderful to have such a kind and patient partner and I'm ashamed to admit that it takes something as drastic as this to make me realize what I have sometimes. I cannot imagine having to deal with this alone, and I know there are women who do.

So I'm just trying to count my blessings, which really are too numerous to even imagine, and to have a thankful heart for all that I do have. On my list of blessings, I count each of you. Thank you for your love, attention and support. I hope you have a great week!!

Love,
Susan

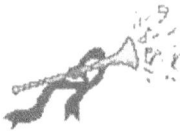

Sunday, June 29, 2003

Good Evening to Everyone!!

We want to thank all of you for your prayers, calls, cards, good thoughts and all the other support we've received from you this week. You are all so kind to remember us and to take time from your lives to let us know you care.

Chemo was Wednesday, and I am cautiously optimistic that we have found a solution for my woes!! I was sick and in the bathroom on Wednesday night, and a little queasy a couple of other times, but the five-day nausea-thon did not appear this time!! I've been able to eat lightly—fruit and dry toast until today, when I ate a half of a tomato sandwich!! How's that for progress??? Other than having a needle left in my port (and therefore my chest) for three days, this experience was a cakewalk compared to last time!!! I did go to the cancer center on Thursday and Friday and get fluids, anti-nausea meds and steroids, and that seems to be the trick for me!! We have been told that we are now 75% complete with the "hard part" of chemo. I've got one more treatment with Adriamycin and Cytoxan on July 15; then we switch to a different chemo agent. We only have five more treatments total left!! It's exciting to see how far we've come!!

I did talk to Dr. Giguere on Wednesday about not being able to retire my razor yet. I told him no one had ever made me look this bad in my whole life, yet still made it necessary for me to shave my legs!!! He told me that when we start Taxol in August, my legs would get smoother!!! Ha—August now seems so far away . . .

I was able to do my Duke torture exercises yesterday, and we are going to walk in a little while, when it gets cooler. Of course, this is my mile an hour pace, but it's good to actually feel like getting out. Our next goal will, of course, be to conquer cardiac hill again before my next chemo. The exercise really seems to be helping my body recover after treatments, and also to help me gather strength to face the next treatments. It may be purely psychological, but I am determined to maintain some sort of exercise routine throughout this regimen.

I have managed to lose 20 pounds since starting chemo, despite being told that I should expect to gain 20-25 pounds. With all the steroids I am receiving, my weight remains a struggle for me. However, I have decided I am stronger than whatever obstacles are placed in my path, and I just have to work with my body to help it recover as quickly as possible from this onslaught. I am amazed anew at the human body and the miraculous way it can continue to renew itself. It's a testament to our Maker that He can create such a fragile, yet robust, work of art.

We have some exciting news to share. Gil has finally decided to have his mid-life crisis and go for a sports car. We are supposed to pick it up tomorrow night—it's an Infiniti G35 Coupe in Caribbean Blue. Gil says I can ride in it, but he's not sure about letting me drive it yet!! :-) Actually, if he isn't nice to me, next year when this is all over and I have been transformed into a babe, I won't ride in it with him!!! Just kidding—of course I'll be able to drive it!!! My husband is so practical and this is such a big step for him. He's been wanting to drive something a little nicer than his pickup truck for a while. God has blessed his company tremendously, and has provided the means for him to have a new toy. So he's going for it!! Congratulations, Gil. And please watch out for the new blue streak driving up and down Highway 25!!!

Our garden is flourishing under Gil's care—we've got baby peppers, tomatoes, squash and cucumbers so far. I just love eating fresh veggies from the garden in the summer. I am not much help this year, except with the weeding on my good days, but I am a tremendous asset when it comes to consumption!! I also do most of the canning and freezing, when our harvest ripens.

I've been enjoying the hummingbird wars on our feeders, and our nesting pair is very charming to watch. The male bluebird is busy, bringing bugs to the female, who faithfully sits on the nest. Soon, they'll both be busy feeding their young. It's wonderful to see life renewed right outside our kitchen window.

We are so blessed to live where we do and to have so much. Gil knows of a lady in the same situation I'm in, who does not have disability insurance, and who is struggling to pay her bills. I am once again humbled to realize how much we take for granted. I heard from my disability insurance company, and they have approved me for benefits until December. I have so much to be thankful for, and yet rarely do I take time to be thankful!! We hope you have a Happy Fourth and a great holiday weekend.

Love,
Susan

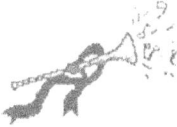

Sunday, July 6, 2003

Hello Everyone!!

As you know, I started feeling better last Sunday, and by Wednesday I felt good. Gil took off work Thursday and Friday for the holiday and we started our day on Thursday by conquering cardiac hill once again. It took a whole hour to walk those two miles, but we did it!! After getting our showers, Gil took me to the Cancer Center Thursday morning. I had only lost four pounds this time—we could all tell the nausea was better!! When I saw Susan, the nurse practitioner, we were both delighted at how my counts had rebounded. She told me to have a great weekend and to enjoy myself for the next week and a half.

Gil and I celebrated by having a late breakfast at Cracker Barrel—one of our very favorite places. We did a few errands, then came home and started mowing. If your grass grows like ours, and if you have had as much rain as we have, you can imagine how long the grass was after not being mowed for three weeks. However, Thursday evening, we managed to break both mowers, and the portable air compressor. We came inside very frustrated, and discovered our basement had at least an inch of water in it!!! So we gave up and went to bed!! When we got up Friday morning, things got better. It's amazing what a good night of sleep will do for you!! Gil managed to fix the riding mower and got the whole yard (remember our yard is five acres) mowed by about 4:30 Friday afternoon.

For July 4, we had a small country celebration at our house with a few friends. Special thanks to Jeff for bringing and manning the grill, Neal and Roxie for rides in the red car, and Linda for photographing the evening for posterity. We had wonderful food, great conversation, and a few small fireworks to top off the evening. Actually, we had four men shooting off the fireworks, and our display lasted about an hour. We had people stopping on our road just to watch!! I think next year we'll charge $5 per carload, just like Furman. (My husband is a closet pyromaniac and he really enjoys his fireworks. He woke up Saturday morning talking about what kind he'll have to get again next year!!!) Seriously, we had a wonderful time celebrating with friends. And we need to have something to look forward to during our "good weeks."

Today Gil took me for a ride in his new car. We went several places we had never been before—Rutherfordton, Spindale and Forest City, NC. Then we rode over to Lake Lure and Chimney Rock and ate ice cream—yum!! The car is a lot of fun and I hope he enjoys it for a long time!!

Tomorrow I see my plastic surgeon again. We haven't done any work on my chest for a month now—things were too stretched the last two times I saw him and it would have been too painful to add any fluid to the expanders. We'll have to see what he thinks tomorrow!!

I have made progress in another area as well. Two weeks ago, I started being able to sleep in bed for the first time since my surgery in early April. For several months, I had been starting out the night in bed, and waking up after 2-3 hours and moving out to the recliner because I was so uncomfortable. Then a couple of weeks ago, I managed to stay in bed for about 5-6 hours before the discomfort woke me up. This past week, it has stretched to 7-8 hours and I am almost able to sleep a whole night now. It's amazing what we take for granted, until it is taken away from us!! I still have to sleep with extra pillows for my arms, and it's a ritual getting me settled, but I'm thankful to be sleeping in a bed again!!

My next treatment is July 15, which is over a week away, and I'm planning to enjoy the coming days. I hope you have a good week—full of everything you enjoy. Summer is a time for friends, fun and relaxing—I hope you are able to have it all!!

Love,
Susan

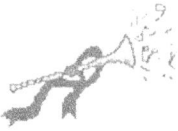

Tuesday, July 22, 2003

Good Morning, Everyone!!!

One week ago today, I had my fourth chemo treatment, and I'm glad it's over!!! I am trying to have a good attitude about chemo, but I find myself dreading the treatments for days before they ever happen!! I was sick in the bathroom before I even left the cancer center this time, and continued to be nauseated and sick until Sunday. However, this was the last of the Adriamycin and Cytoxan, and I'm told that Taxol doesn't have the same gastrointestinal effects as the other two. So, I am celebrating the fact that I am halfway through chemo, and have two weeks until another treatment is due!!! And in just twelve more weeks, I'll be writing to let you know I am completely finished with chemo!! I know it sound like I'm wishing my life away, and I'm trying not to do that. There is so much to be thankful for each day—some days I just have to look a little harder to find it!! I have been asked to correspond with three ladies via e-mail who are all beginning their battle with breast cancer. In particular is a person who is just 36 whose breast cancer has already spread to her bones. She's having a very difficult time with her diagnosis, plus the fact that her disease is so advanced. She's having a lot of pain and fatigue, and it's been a humbling experience for me. It makes me look outside myself and realize how fortunate I am to be diagnosed and treated early in the disease process, and for all the love, care and support we have.

I saw my plastic surgeon two weeks ago and things may have advanced as far as they are going to. The muscles are still very tight over the expanders, so he wants to wait two months and see if any relaxation occurs. If so, he'll fill the expander(s) one more time. If not, I'm not unhappy with my size. Part of my journey this year has been to be thankful for "the little things!!" :-) Seriously, as long as I can buy clothes in a "normal" store, I will be happy!!

I started back on my Duke torture exercises on Sunday—I had hoped to get back to them Friday, but the nausea won out!! It made me very sore Monday, but the exercise really does make a difference in my energy levels and sleeping patterns. I am using the machines inside on "non-Duke" days because I HATE humidity. I'm thankful to have a place to exercise that's safe and comfortable when it's so hot!!!

I did manage to get out in the garden for a short while Sunday night. The tomatoes are turning red, we are harvesting cucumbers daily, and we have a watermelon that will soon be a feast for us!! We are always so ambitious when it comes to planting the garden—we put in 12 tomato plants, and now I wonder why. Just kidding—we made our own tomato sauce last year with fresh tomatoes, peppers and herbs from the garden and it was so good, Gil volunteered to help again this year!!! Gil's corn is about ready to pick—I just love eating fresh veggies from the garden right now!!! We've also had some wonderful peaches lately—there's a little fruit market just up the road and with the wet spring we've had, the peaches are so juicy and good!! Yummy!!

Friday night we're looking forward to seeing Journey and Styx in concert. They are two of my all-time favorite bands from my younger days and are playing in Greenville. We've had tickets since they went on sale in May. My poor long-suffering husband is not a big fan, but this is my belated anniversary present and he's being a very good sport about all this!! We are both old enough now that we're taking earplugs with us!! I don't know if we'll use them, but we'll have them if we need them. I guess that's part of being our 40-something ages—we don't care to have our eardrums ruptured in a single evening anymore!!! But I wouldn't miss this experience for the world!!

If you haven't already heard, Gil has hired a new assistant/ coordinator/ organizer/ woman-of-many-talents to help him. His business has exploded and he's been working many extra hours to try and keep up. He is so pleased with Barbara—she's managed to get his schedule down to manageable and handles many tasks that free him to work with clients. Even though he stays busy with "work outside of work," he's been a much nicer person to be around the past month. We're both pleased that Barbara has been able to relieve some of his burden. They work well together—she's very organized and efficient and has brought order to the chaos of his work life.
Welcome, Barbara—we're both glad you're around!!!

I think that is about it for this time. I hope you have a great week!! Thank you again for all your calls, cards, prayers, gifts and all the ways you show you care!!

Love,
Susan

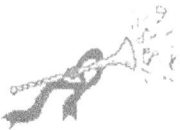

Monday, August 4, 2003

Hello Everyone

It's hard to believe two weeks have already gone by. We have stayed very busy—probably too busy—enjoying life for the past ten days!! We started on

Thursday with swimming, dinner and card games with friends. They are quite the card sharks and Gil and I lost our figurative shirts!! It's a good thing we were only playing for fun. The next day I had my counts done at the cancer center and was told to enjoy my good week.

We went to see Journey, Styx and REO Speedwagon that night. The concert was four hours long and GREAT. Even though we are "old," we still enjoyed ourselves, except for the dancing girls right in front of us. We couldn't see through them and had to stand up a lot, which made me tired, but didn't diminish our fun!! The show started promptly at 7:30 and went until 12:00!! We definitely got our money's worth.

The next day I had a hat party at our house to celebrate being halfway through with chemo. I had 27 girlfriends come over and everyone wore a hat. It was silly, but I still think everyone had a good time. I also got lots of presents—which was totally unnecessary, but delightful, as I LOVE presents. We were supposed to play games, but never got to that because everyone was talking and visiting. Gil and Jackson hid out in his office—I guess it was too much of a hen party for them. I had so much fun that this may become an annual event. And hats off to Brenda for the most wonderful creation to every grace anyone's head—ever!!!

Sunday we went to the movies with friends—we can highly recommend "Seabiscuit" to everyone. What a GREAT movie. After the movie we went out to dinner with our friends and enjoyed visiting with them.

Monday my brother and his wife came for a visit from Houston, TX. This was the first time I had seen my brother since our mother died, almost two years ago. I had never met his wife—she's very sweet and a nice addition to our family. They stayed with us till Wednesday afternoon, and then they left for North Carolina to visit friends. My aunt and uncle from Orlando just happened to be at their second home in Virginia and were traveling back to Orlando on Wednesday, so they came for lunch. And my other aunt, who lives in Asheville, also came for lunch. So we cooked and ate and visited. This was the first time we've had this many of our family together in years—and it was good to see everyone.

Gil actually took two days off last week—thank you Barbara—and on Thursday we went back to the movies. We saw "The League of Extraordinary Gentleman," which is a major guy film, except for one thing—Sean Connery. Gil couldn't believe I liked the movie so much—it's a lot of fantasy and fighting, but with Sean Connery, you can't go wrong!! This was our second movie in one week—we usually don't see two movies in a year, and we are suffering from popcorn overload!!

Friday I had a MUGA scan at the hospital. My ejection fraction was down by 2%, which is a normal amount during chemo. The test is basically a measure of heart function and since both Adriamycin and Taxol can cause myocardial fibrosis (which is stiffening of the heart muscle), it is important to monitor heart function before, during and after chemo. I will have one more
MUGA scan in November, once chemo is over. I did go to the OR and visit—it was nice to see as many people as I did. Everyone told me I didn't look like a chemo patient—I think that's a compliment. I told them if they wanted to see me look sick, they were welcome to come over on Wednesday and see me then!! :-) Seriously, it was good to see friends and catch up on what's going on at work.

Saturday my brother and his wife came back around 5:00 and had dinner with us. They left yesterday morning about 9:00 and got home to Houston at 3:00 their time this morning. They obviously drove straight through—not my kind of trip, but they are home and still have a week of vacation. It was really good to see them and meet David's wife.

Tomorrow I start phase 2 of chemo. I have to take a mega-dose of steroid tonight, another one tomorrow morning before I go to the cancer center. Then, I'll receive even more steroid (I hope I don't end up looking like the Michelin man), Benadryl, Zantac and Anzemet, then the chemo drug Taxol. I'm told Taxol doesn't have near the gastrointestinal effects of the last two drugs. The most common complaint with Taxol is an achy flu-like joint and bone pain. I really hope this is the case. I can lie on the couch and hurt and look really good—as long as I'm not green and nauseated!! I did look Taxol up in my drug book last night and under side effects, it states "60% of patients will have nausea and vomiting."

I just started to cry when I showed Gil. But then I realized that even if I'm sick again, it's only about 20 more rough days, and after tomorrow I'll only have three treatments left!! So it could be worse!! My good friend Brenda is going to be with me tomorrow and I am grateful for her support. I find myself dreading this and have been tense and anxious since yesterday.

I'm working off nervous energy today by cleaning carpets, doing laundry, ironing, etc.—all those things I normally hate to do but getting done today because I can't sit still!! Well, that's about it for us this week. Please remember us in your prayers tomorrow.

I hope you have a great week.

Love,
Susan

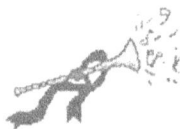

Monday, August 11, 2003

Good Morning!!

What a different experience chemo was this past week!! I certainly don't love Taxol, but I can say good things about it. I am delighted to tell you that I did not have even one minute of nausea or vomiting the whole week. I ate lightly until Friday, anticipating the nausea to show up any second, but it never did!! Hallelujah!! I even had the courage to look in the pantry on Wednesday (the day after chemo)—Gil couldn't believe how brave I was. To celebrate the lack of any stomach complications, on Friday, we had pizza! That's usually a treat that we reserve for late the second week, or even the third week. It was such a relief to get through last week without any gastrointestinal upsets!!

The one "problem" I did have was the achy bone pain. I was fine on Wednesday—just like a normal day (as if I ever have a "normal" day anymore :-)) except for being very tired. I even did my Duke torture exercises Thursday morning—this is usually reserved for at least 5 days post chemo-- and felt quite proud of myself. I started feeling achy on Thursday afternoon— but only from the waist down. My hips and feet were the most affected. By Friday morning, I was hurting everywhere but again, only from the waist down. My little personal pain scale goes: tender, ache, hurt, pain, need medicine. I was to the point of needing Tylenol Friday morning.

I did manage to exercise on the machine, which helped temporarily, as did a blistering hot shower. Gil spent time Friday evening rubbing my feet and legs. By Saturday morning, I was back to achy uncomfortable and mostly in my feet and ankles. Sunday the pain was gone. So if this is going to be my Taxol experience, bring it on!! This means I only have three bad days and six uncomfortable days left! And I have often said that I would rather hurt all over than to be nauseated. So, I will drag out my blanket and lie on the couch and not complain one bit!! I look much better when I'm achy than when I'm green!!

I have also started having hot flashes—ahh, the joys of menopause!! And I'm not even there yet!! It's amazing that in one second my body can change that much. I'll be chilly with a shirt over my tank top, and the next second, I'm pouring sweat and about to roast!! They don't seem to last very long, only about 5-10 minutes and then I'm chilly again!! I never know when they are going to show up either. I wish I could figure out what triggers them, and maybe make an adjustment in what I'm doing. Oh well, if that's all I have to complain about, I really don't have any problems!!

I also have the "wall of fatigue" in front of me right now. Since I felt so good last week, I keep thinking I'm already in my second week post chemo and I shouldn't feel so tired. Ha Ha!! I can do a little project, then I have to sit and rest. I also get breathless very easily, but hey, it hasn't even been a week yet!! I still find naps very refreshing and am enjoying one daily. I wonder when I go back to work, will they allow me an extra hour for a siesta every day??? :-)

We picked over 100 tomatoes on Saturday. Our poor garden has had too much of a good thing—the rain was making the tomatoes split. We also picked peppers, basil, oregano, thyme, sage and chives and made homemade tomato sauce yesterday. It's an all-day project and I was able to sit and rest throughout the day, so it wasn't too hard. Gil also helped and this morning, we took five quarts of tomato sauce out of the pressure canner. It's such a great feeling to grow and can our own produce.

And speaking of Gil, he has finally taken that last step towards becoming a gentleman farmer. Yes, on Saturday, he bought a tractor. It's supposed to arrive either Wednesday or Thursday of this week. When it arrives, he promises to sit on it in a suit and let me get his picture. We'll be sending copies, along with the "Green Acres" theme song. And just to keep in the spirit, our phone number has been changed to BR-549!! :-)

I do have one funny anecdote to share with you. One of Gil's business associates, whom I have not met yet, e-mailed me last week and asked to be added to my list for these updates. He said he wanted to be "kept abreast" of my recovery. I was unaware the he did not know my diagnosis, so of course, I had to ask him exactly what he meant by being kept abreast!! Of course, he was mortified to think he had stepped on my figurative toes. However, I think it's so important to have a sense of humor in life, and was grateful that he made me laugh. I'm looking forward to the day I meet him so he can explain himself!!!

Well, I'm delighted to be able to share some good news with you for a change!! We have received so much support this past week—emails, phone calls, cards, food, volunteers to run errands, etc. I also know there are so many prayer warriors out there and we are always grateful for each of you. Thank you for all the ways you show us you care. May God bless each of you this week!!

Love,
Susan

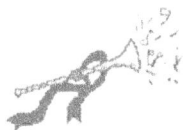

Thursday, August 28, 2003

Hello Again Everyone

I am delighted to tell you that I am now 75% finished with chemo!! YEAH!! I can well remember hearing at the beginning that I would have eight treatments and thinking it would be forever before I was done. I had my sixth treatment Tuesday and there are only two left!! It was a long day at the cancer center, but a successful one. Once again, there has been absolutely no nausea of vomiting and I am so thankful. I think of Kermit the Frog and he spoke very wise words when he sang, "It's Not Easy Being Green!" The fatigue seems to be worse with Taxol and it takes longer to resolve, but I am NOT complaining. I look really good resting on the sofa or recliner, with an afghan over my lap.

I did talk to Dr. Giguere on Tuesday about the bone pain I experienced last time. He asked me to continue taking the steroids until tomorrow and also said I could take some Advil or something with anti-inflammatory properties for these 2-3 days. I did my Duke exercises this morning and started getting a little "achy" shortly afterwards. I popped two Advil, and the ache is hardly noticeable. The only bad side is I have managed to gain eight pounds of steroid weight this week—YUCK!! But I know it will come back off when the drugs are finished. What a difference in this treatment regimen over the last!!

I hope to have my last treatment October 7, and then move on to radiation. Now that I've gotten this far, I really am starting to see that the end is in sight for chemo. There were times that I thought I'd never get done. I understand the principles behind every three weeks, but I am impatient to get past this phase in my life. I was told at the beginning that chemo is a three-week cycle. The first week you feel crummy; the second week you're exhausted and the third week is what everyone looks forward to. And just about the time you start feeling good, it's time for more chemo. I have found this to be true, and it's nice to know I only have to do this two more times. Then I can start feeling good and just "keep going" feeling good.

During my second treatment at the cancer center, my friend Janet and I met a lady who was very inconsistent in her attendance at chemo. Of course, this messes up the regimen and she continually had to "start over" because if she felt good, she just didn't come in for treatment. It could be two or three months between her treatments, instead of three weeks!! At first I was flabbergasted to hear this, but having been through a few rough cycles myself, I can certainly understand her perspective.

When the cooler weather approaches, I am always excited about wearing sweaters and "snuggly" clothes. And since I have all this time off (ha ha), I have been looking at some of the new fall clothes. However, it's going to be different this year. My plastic surgeon is still not finished working on my chest, and nothing really fits right now. I see him again in another week, to see if we are going to be able to do any more expansion on the right side. If so, it will be done before radiation starts. He says I will have to then wait 2-6 months to heal from radiation before he is able to complete his work on my chest. That means a final trip to the operating room to remove the expanders and place the actual implants. I find myself anxious to move on and be done with all this. However, it is a process, not an event and I am thankful that by this time next year, EVERYTHING will be over with, and I'll have my life.

Well, enough about me. Gil had a periodontist visit early in the year and was supposed to have gum surgery in March. Of course, in March is when we found my lump, and things shifted in our universe. We finally got him scheduled and he had his surgery one week ago today. He did remarkably well, and was eating "real" food by Sunday. He only missed work on Friday and was a very good patient. (Of course, I reminded him about paybacks this week, if he didn't behave last week!! :-)) He's still not allowed to eat anything crunchy or hard, like tacos, potato chips, etc., but his mouth looks great. Of course, I attribute this to his excellent in-home nursing care!! And we both want to thank our friend Jodie for providing his anesthesia. She was up almost all night the night before working at the hospital, and still was there for us on Thursday. Gil was very nervous and it made his experience much better knowing she was taking great care of him. Thanks, Jodie—you're the best!!

We are enjoying our garden right now—we're harvesting sweet juicy cantaloupes and watermelons, tasty tomatoes and tons of peppers. There's nothing better than a tomato sandwich on a hot summer afternoon!! And we've had our summer weather the past two weeks. The tomatoes are happy!

It really has been a cool summer by comparison—mostly in the 80s, instead of 90s, and lots of rain. I hear on the weather reports that our fall will be spectacular this year because the leaf stems are so strong from all the rain. Fall is my very favorite time of year, and I always am eager for it to arrive. I can hardly believe this is Labor Day weekend already. In some ways, this summer has dragged, but in others, it has flown by.

Thank you again for all of your calls, cards, food, e-mails and all the other ways you care for us. It's been a challenging time for us, and we are so grateful for all the support we continue to receive from you. Hope you have a great weekend!

Love,
Susan

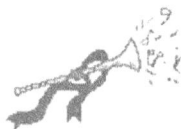

Tuesday, September 9, 2003

Hello Everyone

It's a beautiful afternoon at the beginning of autumn—my FAVORITE time of the year!!! With days like these, you are so thankful to be alive!! Of course, I have a new perspective and am thankful to be alive every day. Our weather in South Carolina just gets prettier every day this time of year. There are a few trees starting to turn colors and we are anticipating a gorgeous fall season for about the next three months!! Yeah!!

Well, I have two more chemo treatments left. The next one is Tuesday of next week. And more importantly, the last one will be four weeks from today. I'm getting very excited. When I started this in May, it seemed like it was going to take FOREVER to get through chemo. I can remember getting the calendar and counting Tuesdays, and marking every third one. I made big stars on Tuesday, October 7.

I understand from the staff at the cancer center that almost everyone who has chemo does this, so I now don't feel quite so strange. When your life revolves around cancer and its treatment, it's hard not to want to "get it over with" and live for the future. There are days when I feel like all I do is take medicine, go see doctors, have blood work done, etc. and deal with this disease. Since I'm on a three-week cycle, we've gotten used to chemo followed by a bad week, then an okay week, then a good week. Just when I start to feel really good, it's time for more chemo!! The nurses also told me this at the beginning of chemo, and said it was very important to enjoy life when I felt good. We have tried to enjoy each day and find beauty in it, but honestly, now that I'm nearing the end of chemo, I can't wait for October 7!!

Most of you know that of all the issues we've faced with breast cancer, I have been the most upset about my hair loss. I am delighted to share that my hair is starting to grow back. Dr. Giguere keeps telling me that it will all come out with Taxol (the chemo drug I'm receiving now), but I've had two treatments, and I haven't seen any hair on my pillow. And believe me, I'm checking every day!! Last time I had chemo I asked him if I was getting enough of the drug since I had hair on my head!! I wasn't trying to criticize, but I would hate for them to tell me I didn't get enough chemo and have to have more. Especially after October 7!!

Dr. Giguere said my hair would feel like a puppy when it first started growing back, and it does. Unfortunately, it is coming is gray instead of brown. Oh well, I've been a "bottled brunette" for years, and I am NOT complaining about any color hair at this point. Several of my friends have tried to express to me their frustration with bad hair days this past summer, and I just have no sympathy for them!! :-)

I'm actually looking forward to bad hair days again!! Dr. Giguere also says that my eyelashes and eyebrows will come out with Taxol. I lost about half of them with the first dose of Adriamycin, and they have stayed thin, but present, since. It takes me about 10 minutes to put on enough mascara that it looks like I have eyelashes, but at least I do still have them. So maybe I'm going to get my hair early. I'm terribly excited about it and hopeful this is really the start of the re-growth!! And in case you're wondering, yes, I am STILL shaving my legs!!!

I saw my plastic surgeon yesterday and he said we were through with expansion. He tells me I have to wait 2 to 6 months post radiation for my body to heal before he can do anything else for me. I'm voting for two months. Since I don't finish radiation until the end of December, the earliest appointment I could have was late February. Then I'll have one more surgery to remove these very uncomfortable tissue expanders and place the breast implants. I don't think I'll ever be able to work at Platinum Plus (our local strip club in Greenville), but that was never one of my goals anyway!! Now, February seems so far away.

With our beautiful weather starting this past weekend, Gil and I walked Sunday morning for the first time in six weeks. It was wonderful to be outside and to once again conquer cardiac hill. I walked again this morning—my speed was a 15-minute mile and it felt great. Even though I have been exercising inside during the worst of the humidity, I am sore from working those leg and rear end muscles on the hill.

With the high dose steroids I'm taking, I have gained back 14 pounds! I still am 9 pounds less than when I started chemo, but I also have two more treatments with those same high dose steroids. It is frustrating to look at those numbers on the scale, but I am not giving up. I have to realize that it is an induced weight gain and it will go away again once the drugs are finished.

It will be nice to work in the yard again soon. We planted milkweeds for the monarch butterflies last year, with no visitors. We replanted them again this year and we saw monarch butterflies all over them in August. Well, they obviously laid eggs because we are now watching the caterpillars eat the bushes to the ground! We even have one caterpillar inside in a jar, so Gil can watch the whole process of caterpillar-cocoon-butterfly. He's never seen it from start to finish and we're eagerly anticipating the process!!

Gil's mouth has healed nicely from his oral surgery. Dr. Hamrick told him last week to eat whatever he wanted (I wish a doctor would tell me that!! :-)) and come back in a month. He still can't use the electric toothbrush for eight weeks, but other than that, he's healed! Thank you for asking about him—he did great, thanks to his wonderful in-home postop nursing care!! :-) By the end of the year, we should both be healthy and ready for a new year!! That's about it from us in Tigerville. I hope you're having a good week. Thank you for your cards, e-mail, food, prayers and support.

Love,
Susan

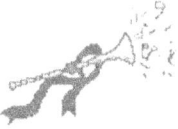

Wednesday, September 24, 2003

Good Morning Everyone

It's a beautiful autumn morning and at the risk of repeating myself again, I LOVE this time of year. I just finished walking and I was so thankful for the lower humidity and the ability to walk outdoors again. The trees in our area are starting to turn colors and I think it just gets prettier and prettier with every passing day. I saw "our" twin fawns while walking—they are getting big and losing their spots. Their mother has sent them on their way—they are always together now, but without her. They were in our woods Sunday and Monday and when they came bounding across the grass, we just had to stop everything and watch them for a minute. They are very skitterish and don't stay long, but it's wonderful to see them when they're around.

Chemo #7 was last week and went as well as it can. I'm still not having any nausea and am able to eat almost anything, starting the next day. And I do!! The "Period of Aches and Yucks" lasted from Thursday to Sunday this time. The extra steroids and Advil are helping diminish the bone pain quite significantly, but I still think I look really good lying on the couch with a blanket!! By yesterday, I started feeling good again. Now it's the "Wall of Fatigue," but that's nothing to complain about. I just have to have lots of rest periods throughout the day. When I feel this good, it's easy to get going on a project and not rest when I should. Then I really pay for it the next day!!

I was able to do my Duke exercises last Thursday (2 days post-chemo), which is the earliest ever. I was very shaky and sweaty (is this too much info?) and it took me twice as long as usual because I had to sit down between sets, but I was very proud of myself for getting up and moving!!

On Friday, I walked up cardiac hill—remember the hill that's about 3/10 mile straight up? I won't say I conquered it because I had to stop and breathe four times on the way up, but I did make it to the top. Today I managed to make it up the hill, stopping only once, and go a little farther as well.

Our addresses out here change at the one-mile mark, so I can proudly boast that I walked to Landrum this morning!! It took me over an hour, but every day it will get a little easier again. Poor Jackson feels like he's walking with a little old lady. He goes a little ahead, then stops and waits. Even though he can't fully understand, he's very patient with the pace right now. The exciting part is that I only have to recover from chemo one more time and the walk will be much easier.

I can tell my counts have dropped. I get breathless very easy and have to rest after just a little exertion. It is amazing how much one part of your body can affect all the rest of the body. When I went for chemo last week, Dr. Giguere himself told me that my counts were so consistently recovering that I didn't have to come in this week at all!! He said to have a good three weeks and he would see me October 7. Of course I didn't argue. I have gotten to where I hate even driving into the parking lot at the cancer center. And I don't have to get any needles until two weeks from now. Yeah!!

My hair re-growth continues and I am thrilled. I did pull off my bandana and show Dr. Giguere my hair last week. I asked him again if I was getting enough chemo drugs and he said yes. I am also starting to "sprout" hair in other places that have been naked this summer. Dr. Giguere said I should be prepared for a great "molt" before my final hair comes in. I hope not. What I have is very soft and fine. It's not long enough to curl yet, but I'm hoping for curls! It's kind of like Christmas and wondering what's inside that package under the tree!! I can say that whatever color and texture it is, I will be thankful for hair every day when I look in the mirror!! And yes, I'm looking forward to bad hair days again!!! Working in the OR and wearing a hat doesn't make for pretty hair, but that's also going to be something to appreciate again!!

Remember me telling you about our caterpillar? He became a cocoon two weeks ago today. We've been watching the beautiful emerald green chrysalis darken and yesterday it became transparent. You can actually see the butterfly's wings now—there is orange with black veining and white spots visible through the walls of the cocoon. We've had monarchs floating around our yard all week. We'd like to think they are siblings of "our" butterfly that hatched a little earlier. And "our" butterfly will have companionship on the migration. They are so beautiful to watch and we have enjoyed them all summer. With the cooler weather comes changes—and even though I love the weather, I will miss the butterflies and hummingbirds.

Our local Susan G. Komen walk is this Saturday. We are hoping to go and watch the start of it. Next year, I will be contacting each of you for your support. My friends have decided that we are all going walk in our hats and raise money for breast cancer research, and then we'll go have our second annual hat party! I think that sounds like lots of fun, but I want everyone to remember the purpose of the walk and the women who have and will battle breast cancer.

We are planning on working outside in the yard over the next two weeks. We have seriously neglected the flowerbeds and have a wonderful crop of crabgrass. With Gil being Dutch, we always plant lots of bulbs in the fall. It's fun to go get the bulbs, but when we get home, we always ask, "Why did we buy so many? Where are we going to put them?" But in the spring, we are glad again!! It's been in the lower 40s at night at our house several times. So I think it's time for bulbs, pansies and mums.

Well, I hope you're able to enjoy fall as much as I do. It's been a challenging year, and I'm glad to see it getting further behind us. I hope you have a great week!!

Love,
Susan

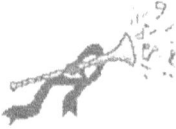

Wednesday, October 8, 2003

Good Morning Everyone

I am ecstatic to report that I have finished chemotherapy!!! Yesterday was my last treatment and I now have all eight of them behind me. For the past two days, Gil and I have been saying to each other, "we're going to (unmentionable place) for the last time." What a great feeling it is to be finished with such a challenging and difficult time. Gil was with me yesterday and the day went rather quickly. I also had visits AND presents from two very special friends. Thank you Janet and Danette!! We were out of the cancer center by 2:30 and had lunch at the Olive Garden to celebrate. I still can't get over the fact that I can eat like a normal person during this time, but I'm not holding back!! I still take Anzemet for nausea for three days post-chemo. I haven't had any nausea with Taxol, but I'm also not taking any chances!!

This was also the last time for the high-dose steroids. I will still take them today, tomorrow and Friday, but that's it! And I am delighted with myself for not gaining any additional weight. I was down a net five pounds yesterday from my starting weight. I have put back on 18 pounds, but still weigh less than when I started. I can remember being told that the average chemo patient can expect to gain 23 pounds during treatment and I made up my mind at the beginning that it wasn't going to happen to me. As someone who has struggled with weight issues my whole life, I am very proud of this accomplishment. In addition to finding out I had breast cancer in March, I also learned that my cholesterol and triglycerides were VERY high. These values have been monitored over the summer and I have managed to lower my triglycerides by over 200 points. That alone proves I have been exercising, even though my weight continues to be artificially elevated from the steroids. But this was a great boost for me continuing to exercise. Now with the steroids almost finished, I hope the weight will come off as well. Gil and I were up to walking five miles this past weekend, at pretty normal pace for us. We did it in an hour and 20 minutes, and were very pleased. I plan to start the Duke exercises back tomorrow and walking on Friday again. Of course, it will take me an hour to walk two miles, but that's how it starts. And it's exciting to know that now when I build back up to my distance and speed this time, it will be FOR THE LAST TIME!!!

We did go to the Susan G. Komen walk two Saturdays ago. What a wonderful experience for anyone who is, or knows someone who is, battling breast cancer. It was a warm and humid morning, so I only wore a bandana (on my head, in addition to my other clothes—I know how your minds work!) and there were many women coming up to me and telling me their stories and how many years of survival they had achieved. It was so encouraging to have that support and realize that I will be there too!! We watched the start of the races and were surprised how many men were participating. There were several white doves released just before the starting bell and instead of flying off somewhere, they flew in circles the runners. I stood there with tears streaming down my face in amazement and gratitude that I was able to be present for such an exciting event. Now more than ever, I am planning on participating next year. I called one of my friends that Saturday night and asked if she had watched the story on the news. She said she had and then said, "We ARE going to be walking next year, not running, right?"

I did have some disappointing news this past week. My hospital apparently has a policy that neither my bosses nor I were aware of that states any employee who is out on medical leave past six months must be terminated. So last Friday, I lost my job. I have been told that I am eligible for re-hire and that in January, when I can return to work, I have should re-apply. I asked about my five-year anniversary that had occurred just before I received my diagnosis in March, and have been assured by Human Resources that those milestones will be honored. It was very discouraging to hear this news just seven days before it was supposed to happen, but to put things in perspective, once you've been told you have cancer, you can deal with just about anything else. And I do believe God's hand is upon this whole episode in my life, and that He has a plan. Now, if I can be patient and recognize this fact, I will be just where I need to be in January.

I next see Dr. Giguere on October 28 and will start taking tamoxifen for five years. This is an anti-estrogen drug. Since my tumor was very positive for estrogen and progesterone receptors, this hormone will work to kill any estrogen in my body. If this doesn't work, I am told that I will have to have my ovaries removed surgically. They want me to have absolutely no estrogen produced ever again. I think by the end of all this, I will be almost completely androgynous!! Then it's on to radiation. I will hopefully start the first week of November and have 30 to 35 treatments. I haven't met the radiation oncologist yet, but hear they are both very nice men. I was also reassured again yesterday that after chemo, radiation is a "piece of cake." I should finish this just before Christmas. Then this whole challenging and difficult year will be behind us. The start of the new year will be like a new life for us. And I am glad to be here for it!!

We certainly have appreciated each of you and all the support we've received. Having a cancer diagnosis gives you a whole new perspective and makes you very thankful for so many things. It has been so encouraging to us to know how many friends we have and to learn to slow down and enjoy life a little more. Thank you for all the ways you each have ministered to us. We are so blessed to have so many wonderful people in our lives.

I hope you have a great week!!

Love,
Susan

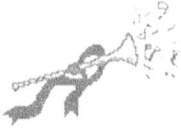

Wednesday, October 29, 2003

Hello Everyone

I saw Dr. Giguere yesterday and for the first time in 24 weeks, did not have to have more chemo!! I am still realizing it is finally over!! He said my counts looked great and that I was now a "graduate." He prescribed Tamoxifen for me, which I will take daily for the next five years. It is an anti-estrogen hormone, so if my body is still producing estrogen, this should shut it off. If not, there are other drugs, and if that doesn't work, there is surgery!! They drew additional blood to check ovarian function and I will have lab results at my next visit in late November to see what is going on inside my body. My tumor had receptors on it that were very estrogen and progesterone positive. Since this is what helped the breast cancer start, I cannot have any more estrogen for the rest of my life. Now if my voice deepens, and I grow facial and chest hair, you know why!! A small trade-off when you consider I also won't have breast cancer either!!

I had some very exciting news yesterday. For those of you who don't know about the magic five years, once you have been diagnosed with cancer and had surgery, chemo, radiation, etc. to eradicate the cancer, the next five years are very important. When you get to your five-year anniversary and have remained cancer free, you are considered "normal" again. You can get insurance without a pre-existing condition being considered, you can donate blood, etc. It is almost like you never had cancer. Well, I asked if my five-year countdown could now begin, since I was finished with chemo. And Dr. Giguere said I had started mine in April, with surgery. So I am already half a year towards that magic number. My five-year anniversary date will be April 5, 2008!!

I have an appointment on November 6 with Dr. Jeannette Wilcox, who is a radiation oncologist. Several of you have asked why I will be having radiation, since I've already had chemo. Dr. Giguere said that one to three positive lymph nodes is questionable for radiation, but since I had four positive nodes, I am definitely going to have it. Additionally, he told me since I was so young (can you see why I like him so much??), I was getting a "double whammy" with chemo and radiation. Hopefully, we'll get my chest marked and everything in order next week so I can start radiation the following week. I like having a woman doctor, since we are dealing with my chest. Although there isn't much to see now, it's still my chest!! Meanwhile, I have eight days off to "play" and am looking forward to enjoying our beautiful fall weather. It has finally gotten cool here—it feels like October now!!

I also want to thank Ann Geier for making me feel very special. She is our local AORN president and in her message to our chapter last week, she talked about my story. She started off by calling me a breast cancer survivor!! This is the first time I have been referred to as a survivor and as I read her message, I was overwhelmed and just sat and shed tears of joy. The summer has been such an emotional time—with very high highs and very low lows. Although I have never doubted I would make it to this point, it was so wonderful to see it in print, and realize it HAS happened. Thank you, Ann!!

We had our annual Halloween party last Saturday night. In addition to Halloween, we were also celebrating the end of chemo. Since we have been married, Gil and I have never dressed up for Halloween, but this year was different. He was Tonto and I was Chemo-sabe. Part of my costume included a small stuffed white horse with a hot pink mane and tail. She was also decorated and had blue eye shadow, silver false eyelashes, pink blush and red lipstick. If you haven't guessed, she was 'Ho Silver. We have pictures "in the camera," and when we get them printed, I'll share them with you. We had a great time and it's so wonderful to have our friends help celebrate the end of such a challenging summer.

We have so many reasons to be thankful and I count each of you as one of them!! We have been so blessed by your support and I am grateful.

I hope you have a great week!!

Love,
Susan

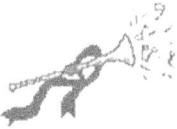

Thursday, November 13, 2003

It's a chilly, windy Thursday afternoon in Upstate South Carolina . . . it seems like fall has arrived with a bang!! Our temperatures are supposed to be in the 20s tonight, and I think Gil may even turn on the heat, though it isn't December yet!!! :-) My Canadian husband enjoys the cool weather, but we're actually competing this year to see who can tolerate the lower temperatures better. It looks like I'm winning, thanks to my hot flashes!!

I met with Dr. Wilcox last week and really liked her. I had another complete History and Physical and we discussed the process of radiation. She told me that, with surgery and radiation, I was completely cancer free at this point. However, I had a 40% chance of recurrence without radiation. I was shocked to hear this, and she hastened to assure me that I also had a 60% chance of no recurrence. Those numbers were awfully close to 50-50 and I found that really scary. Then she went on to explain that with radiation, that 40% chance can be decreased to a 10% chance of recurrence. So obviously, I opted to undergo radiation. Gil also pointed out that breast cancer occurs in 1 in every 8 women, which is 12.5%, so my chances are now less than "the average woman."

The good news about all this is that I only have to have 25 treatments, instead of 35, like we originally thought. Since I had a full mastectomy and have no breast tissue left, Dr. Wilcox said I only needed 25 exposures. I also do not have to have my axilla radiated, and that was a bonus. She said since 11 lymph nodes had been removed, and only the first four were positive for tumor cells, surgery was considered curative in that area. So we went to the treatment area and I spent almost an hour in a CT scanner. Dr. Wilcox used my mammogram films and the operative notes from Dr. Bour to determine where my tumor had been. There are lasers throughout the room and between the computer and Dr. Wilcox's calculations, the table I was on was moved and rotated and was raised and lowered to line up my chest in the crosshairs of the lasers to get precise markings. Then my right chest was painted with black and blue body paint, which was all covered with tape. I was told to come back Wednesday (yesterday) for the actual treatments to begin.

Since they want to be really precise with the radiation, we repeated this whole process yesterday. Then I was placed in a radiation simulator. We spent about 45 minutes re-checking and painting with purple and black marks yesterday. They also used the simulator to make plates, which fit in a slot between me and the "radiator" part of the machine. These plates shield my thyroid and other important structures that aren't supposed to receive any treatment. I wonder if they're made from Kryptonite. Hmmm.

Then I walked over to the treatment room. In this room, the patient lays on a table that can go up and down, and rotate 180 degrees in each direction. The actual machine that delivers radiation is huge, and hums all the time. It forms a big "C" around the person, and the whole C has 360 degree movement. The table I was on moved back towards the machine and the machine moved toward me simultaneously. I laid on my back, and my right arm got placed in a holder that keeps it out and up towards my head. I am also supposed to hold my head like I'm looking over my left shoulder. There are more lasers in this room, so my chest was lined up with a red grid. All of a sudden, the C part of the machine appeared over my head and it was very close. It was humming and spinning and whirring the whole time. There were three technicians running the machine, the computer, and double-checking angles and measurements. Then someone says, "Here we go," and all the technicians leave the room.

The machine hummed louder and all of a sudden it started beeping—that's when it's actually delivering the radiation. I have three "shots" from three different angles. So as soon as it is finished with one burst, the machine started moving and humming and the table moved to re-position for the next shot. Even though I was looking at a fixed point to try and keep my bearings, it was kind of like being inside a gyroscope!! I was told that it takes more time to set up for each shot than it does to actually deliver the radiation. The actual bursts of radiation are probably less than 20 seconds; it just seems like they last forever!!

I went back for a second treatment today, and things were a little more familiar. I am still in an unknown world and while it is impressive, it is also intimidating and frightening. There has been a feeling of vulnerability throughout this whole treatment process, and being the control freak that I am, I don't like it!! This is a very high tech process and I think if I weren't the patient, this would be a fascinating experience!! I will go to radiation every day the cancer center is open, including the day after Thanksgiving. This puts me on track to finish December 17!! So a new countdown has begun!!

The side effects from radiation aren't nearly as severe as from chemo. Dr. Graham told me earlier, and Dr. Wilcox reminded me, of the possibility of capsular contracture—which is when the tissue surrounding the tissue expander "shrinks" from the radiation and "clamps down" around the expander. Yesterday as I was walking out of the cancer center, my right chest already felt tighter and harder. And today, it was even more pronounced. If things keep up at this rate, I'll have a lethal weapon to use when I hug someone!! The other common side effect I was told to expect was a skin burn, which is like a really bad sunburn. My skin is pink and very warm (and is just what I needed to go with my hot flashes!!!) and I'm using aloe gel on it daily. But if this is all there is, I think I can handle it. Radiation is still WAY better than chemo!!

I also completed my 6 month Duke study yesterday. I get to keep all the "toys" including the torture ball. My sweet husband told me my hips and thighs look smaller and that he thinks these exercises have made a difference. I don't need any more motivation to keep doing these exercises, even though the official program is complete. It's been a challenge and I still hate cardiac hill, but the MUGA scan I had last week showed a significant improvement in my heart functioning!! YEAH!! Special thanks to Beth at Duke, who has been a cheerleader, an encourager and a wonderful source of support.

Well, that's enough about me. I appreciate all your calls and questions about radiation and how we're doing, and I hope I've been able to help answer most of them. I can't believe that November is almost half over. As we approach Thanksgiving, Gil and I want to thank each of you for all the support you have given us this year. With our families being so far away, we have relied on our friends, and each of you has blessed us. Every request has been met with kindness and compassion. And we've had so many wonderful surprises along the way. I have so much to be thankful for, and each of you is on my list of blessings. I hope you have a wonderful Thanksgiving holiday.

Love,
Susan

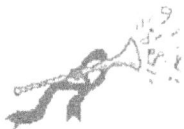

Friday, December 19, 2003

Greetings to everyone!!!

I hope you're well on your way to being ready for the holidays, because ready or not, here they come!!! I finished our Christmas cards this morning and Gil is mailing them, along with our last two packages today. Yippee!!! Now I can get into some serious baking. It's cookie time in our house. I've been to BJ's (our local warehouse store) and Publix and bought all the flour, sugar, butter, chocolate chips, nuts, etc. to make some serious cookies. I am so looking forward to doing this--it's a lot of work, but I LOVE it and I have missed out on too much this year. I have several girlfriends coming over tomorrow to help. A couple of girls started this several years ago, and it's becoming a tradition. We started out having cookie night, now we have cookie weekend!! We make 12 kinds of cookies to share. If you're in the area, feel free to stop by and have a sample. Our house always smells so good this time of year!!

I've heard from lots of you wanting to know how radiation is going. Well, I thrilled to report that it is going, going, GONE! I finished my last treatment yesterday! After 25 sessions with "that machine," I am done!! When I got out to my car yesterday, I realized that ALL the treatments are finally finished and I just started screaming!!! Then I called Gil and we screamed together. It was such a joy to know I've taken all that can be done and I don't have to take anymore!!!

I was told that after chemo, radiation was a piece of cake. Well, I wouldn't call it cake exactly, but it did turn out to be easy to do and I didn't get sick, which was a huge blessing. Dr. Wilcox told me I had sailed through it. I do have a pretty painful burn under my arm and on my chest. I'm using aloe, Desitin and another ointment, wearing soft old T-shirts and taking Tylenol.

For about the last week of my treatments, I had blisters that popped and even though my skin was burned and sore, the radiation continued. It wasn't fun to have fresh, tender skin get burned, but that's part of it. Dr. Wilcox said the discomfort would probably continue for about a week, and then it would get much better quickly. I will probably peel, and I'm sure my skin won't look the same again, but the important thing is I am cancer free!!! I'm hoping to feel better by Christmas Day. And in the big picture, I am very fortunate. This week I met a lady who is in her early 50s who has inoperable brain tumors. She is receiving chemo and radiation together and they are hoping to shrink her tumors, but her cancer cannot be cured. Any time I want to feel sorry for myself, I just have to go to the cancer center.

I also met another lady who was diagnosed with Stage 4 (supposedly terminal) breast cancer in 1996. It had gone into her lymph nodes and she had metastases on her brain, ribs, lungs, pelvis and several other places. She went through chemo and radiation and is cancer free today. What an inspiration she was for me. We talked about how advanced the treatments we receive today are compared to 10 or 25 years ago, then we laughed at how barbaric they will seem in 10 to 25 years. She told me she has never felt free from her cancer and that it is something she lives with every day. I don't know if the worries will ever go away completely, but I'm certainly planning on putting all this behind me and moving on to LIFE again.

I will see Dr. Wilcox in mid-January for a skin check and Dr. Giguere in February for a checkup. I have already graduated to seeing Dr. Giguere every three months. This goes for two years, and then I'll see him every four months for another year. Then it's every six months for two more years, then annually. It's a little scary to be released from all this structure and schedule I've been following, but also very liberating. I am so thankful to be on this side of the treatment process. I'm even more thankful to know that my diagnosis was made early in the disease process and that I am cured. We can certainly see God's hand on us throughout all this.

I want to thank you for all your encouragement this year--at the beginning of this (way back in March), someone sent me an e-mail that said, "Friends are angels that carry us when our wings have forgotten how to fly." Our wings were very sad earlier this year, yet we never felt alone. You have all been such a constant and abiding source of comfort, love and support. We could not ask for better friends and we are so grateful to you for your prayers, love and concern. I hope each of you have a wonderful Christmas--we're celebrating a little extra this year!!

I'm ready to put 2003 behind me, and am looking for wonderful things for all of us in 2004!!!

Merry Christmas!!

Love,
Susan

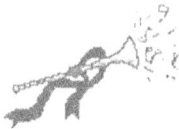

Monday, January 26, 2004

Hello Everyone

So many of you have been asking when I will write another update. Since this 2004 has begun, I haven't been dealing with cancer on a daily basis and have gotten slack in my writing!! However something happened that I want to share with you. One of my good friends from high school has offered to make a memory book for me detailing our lives last year. She wanted to include meaningful e-mails not only between the two of us, but others that had touched me throughout last year. I have just finished re-reading them and am once again awestruck and humbled by the love and support we received from so many people last year. I have saved every e-mail because they are precious to me and there are over 600 of them!!! My friend didn't realize what she was getting herself into when she offered to do this for me!! Her inbox will be overloaded with e-mail from my forwards this afternoon and I am eagerly anticipating the "book" she is making for me. While reading the e-mails again, I have laughed, cried, and experienced so many emotions—what a blessing they were to us in such a horrific time in our lives. But with the New Year, we realized that life has started anew, without the specter of breast cancer and its treatment hanging over our heads!!

As you know, I had my last radiation treatment on December 18. I was told the burn would continue to worsen for "a couple of weeks." That proved to be very true and I was thankful I had only received 25 treatments, instead of 35!!! The skin actually turned black in places and sloughed in big patches. It was quite painful and very disgusting as well!! I was wearing old t-shirts and tank tops and changed tops 5-6 times a day!! I think Christmas day was the worst; then I began to get progressively better. By the 14th day (New Year's Day), I was almost healed and just felt tender in that area. Now I have a lovely radiation "tan"—I still don't understand why I couldn't just lay out in the sun and accomplish the same results ☺--and my skin is not painful at all. I am wearing "normal" clothes and looking forward to getting on with my life!!

Gil and I did get to go on a road trip and had a great time. The same friend who is making my memory book invited us to her daughter's wedding on December 27 in Eclectic, Alabama. Bear in mind that we both grew up in Tampa, Florida and graduated from high school 25+ years ago (does that make us OLD friends?) and throughout the years and moves, we have managed to stay in touch. Gil and I decided the morning of December 26 that I felt well enough to travel, if Gil did most of the driving. So we took our goats to a friend's house for the week and got a wonderful neighbor to baby-sit our house and chickens for us. We packed our clothes, the car, the dog's accessories and left Saturday morning. It was a five-hour drive to Eclectic, which we made without any trouble. We even had time to rest in the hotel for about an hour before the wedding started. The wedding was wonderful and we stayed after to help undecorate the church and get it ready for Sunday morning services. We then went back to our friends' house and talked forever---isn't it amazing how you can just pick up where you left off ten years ago, like it was yesterday? Sunday morning we went to breakfast with our friends, and then Gil and I continued our trip to Pensacola, Florida for the next few days. Our hotel room was right on the beach and it was awesome. We kept the door open so we could hear the waves the whole time!!! It was about 75 degrees during the day, low humidity and PERFECT weather. It was also practically deserted and we had the beach pretty much to ourselves. We spent our days walking on the beach, reading, napping, playing tourists, and eating—the perfect vacation!!

We started home on New Year's Day and drove through Tallahassee. Even though I am a Florida native, I am embarrassed to admit that I had never been to the state capitol before. We also got to tour the Florida State campus (go 'Noles) and it was a great time because everyone else was in Miami for the Orange Bowl. We drove the back roads of Georgia until after dark—Gil had never seen the countryside and we HAD to get some boiled peanuts!! It was quite scenic and peaceful and a lovely drive.

We spent the night in Forsyth—a little south of Atlanta. Since the Peach Bowl was being played on January 2 in Atlanta, we continued our journey home on more of Georgia's back roads. I think we saw every cow in Northeast Georgia and I can attest to the fact that none of them were acting "mad." We did get to stop in Commerce and do a little shopping at the outlet mall there. Then we continued home and had a wonderful weekend. As you know, it is often difficult for Gil to take any time off work, but he said he could do this same trip every year at this time—how's that for a tribute to the wonderful time we had!!

I saw Dr. Wilcox on January 15 and she has discharged me from her care. That means I am completely healed from the radiation and ready to resume a "normal" life. I am very thankful she was my radiation oncologist—she is very kind and caring and genuinely cares about her patients. She hugged me and told me she was available if I needed anything, and I hugged her back and told her I hoped I never saw her again!! At least while she is at work!!

I did get to meet one of my e-mail breast cancer buddies and have breakfast with her. A mutual friend asked me to share my story with her, and we began exchanging e-mails last June. She was a few weeks behind me in her diagnosis and treatment schedule, and it worked out that the day I saw Dr. Wilcox, she was having radiation near the same time and we arranged to meet face-to-face. She is a beautiful woman named Hope and it was wonderful to sit down and share with each other. No matter how supportive someone is, they just can't understand like someone who has been through what you've endured. I hope we'll continue to stay in touch now that this is behind both of us.

I will see Dr. Graham in mid-February and am VERY excited about undergoing my final surgery with him. I have had these tissue expanders in my chest since last April and they have never been comfortable. The right side has a contracture around the expander from the radiation and hurts all the time. This is a very small complaint, compared to what I see and hear every time I go to the cancer center. I am very eager to have my implants placed and heal one last time. I think once I have this last surgery, it will finally bring closure to this episode.

I did re-apply at the hospital and contacted my old bosses about a position with the hospital, and was told there are no positions in the OR at this time. I was ready to go back to work, so I initially felt very discouraged and frustrated, but then realized that God has closed those doors, for whatever reason. In the past, when I've beaten and pounded on God's closed doors, often when I got to the other side of the door, I realized I didn't want to be there anyway. So I am praying for patience and grace to handle this situation. And for now, I plan to stay home and continue to rest and heal. I have energy to do what I want, but not stamina to go for long periods. We are continuing to have a large payment to the hospital for our COBRA insurance (which at this point I cannot be without), but I have so much to be thankful for. Fortunately, Gil makes enough money to pay all our bills and we will be fine. I realize that this isn't the case for many people, and it's just one more area that I realize how we are provided for every day.

I hope the year has started off well for each of you. This time last year, we had no idea what was in store for us in 2003, and I could not have imagined it in my wildest dreams. It is soooooooooo great to be on this side of things and to be able to look back and find the good in each day. I wish you happiness, peace, and love this year. May God bless each of you!!

Love,
Susan

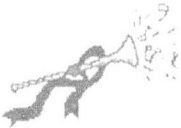

Sunday, February 29, 2004

Happy Leap Day Everyone!!

I'm writing the last chapter in my update journal to you today. I had my final surgery on Friday and yes, I now have boobs, instead of boob-lets. I have just had a shower and am wearing an actual bra for the first time since last May!! I never thought I would look forward to wearing a bra, but it actually feels comfortable!! The incisions and drain sites are "stinging" and my entire chest is sore, but I've only taken Tylenol, except at night, since Friday!! Dr. Graham "lowered" everything on my chest and I actually look more "normal" than I have for the past year. But more importantly, he released the capsular contracture on the right side that has been so painful since radiation. When I woke up in recovery, I could already feel that the constant pressure and pain that has been a part of my life for almost a year was gone!! Hallelujah!! Gil has been impressed with what I can already do and says he thinks I'm already about where I was two weeks post-op last year. He's having to do lifting and reaching for me, but I'm surprised at how much independence I have already. I also had my port (for vascular access) removed on Friday, and that incision is hurting the most!! It will be a couple of weeks before I can hop and jump, but I can see and feel a huge improvement, even with the swelling I've got now!! A very special thanks to Sherry, Reynette, Becky and Sally for their excellent care and for making this as easy as possible for me at the hospital.

Just as exciting was the news I received from Dr. Giguere on February 17. I had my first three-month follow up visit with him then and he said I looked very healthy and that I should continue doing everything I had been doing. He gave me a physical and said I had the best pair of lungs he had heard this year. He asked what I was doing and I told him I had been walking and he said to keep it up! He said there is still no evidence of the cancer's return and that he would see me in May. We were discussing how long this has been going on and realized that we found my lump on March 7 and I was told I had breast cancer on March 27. So it's been almost a year. Everyone tells me how fast it has gone, but I don't feel that way. I do feel like I have not just finished the last chapter in a very long book, but actually closed the cover of the book. And it's a book I never want to pick up again. We are very cognizant of the fact that this could recur at any time, but I am so optimistic about my doctors' decisions and the success of the treatments. And it has taught us not to waste a single minute of life. It really is just too short to squander.

As you may remember, my hair was my biggest issue last year. I am pleased to tell you it has grown to about two and a half inches long and I have curly tips on it. It is pretty much doing what it wants and every day is a bad hair day to me, but I am not complaining!! I took my wigs back to the wig store on Monday--where they will be cleaned and donated to the American Cancer Society. They were still in good shape and I hope someone who really needs them will get good use from them. As I walked out the door and got in my car, I just burst into tears--realizing this year is finally over!!

I also have a funny story about my hair. It's long enough now that I don't look like a chemo patient anymore. I was at our veterinarian's office in October with my Halloween bandana and we talked about chemo. I was back in the office this past week with our new puppy (more on that in a minute) and after she examined the puppy and gave her shots, etc., she asked me who cut my hair. I was so taken aback, I just said, "What?" She said, "You have a great style. Who does your hair?" I just started laughing and she asked me why that was a funny question. I then told her this was my chemo hair and it hasn't been cut by anyone, and in fact, I'm not cutting it for a long time!! (Actually, May 12 is one year ago that I got it cut off, and I already have an appointment for my first cut.) It was so exciting to realize yet again that "hell" year really is over!!!

Now, about the new puppy. She's a stray--remember we live out in the country and many people take this as an invitation to drop off unwanted pets. Our neighbors--Jeff and Julie--found her at their end of our road, caught in the bushes. They already have seven dogs--most adopted strays, and just couldn't handle another one. So this one was headed to the pound. Julie put out "found dog" signs all over and no one claimed her. And my soft-hearted husband said she just couldn't go to the pound. The vet says she is about five months old, part Jack Russell terrier, part rat terrier, with some hound (probably beagle) mixed in. We're calling her Sadie and she's just adorable. We have some work to do with house-training, etc., but we really think she's going to be a great dog. She's mostly white, with reddish brown spots. She's only about 20 pounds and is a good-size indoor dog. Jackson thinks she's his dog and they are both adapting to each other really well. They play for hours at a time and it's good entertainment for us. She's still very uncoordinated and "tumbly" when she runs or plays, and we're having lots of fun watching her.

I still haven't heard anything about a job at the hospital. I wasn't really ready to actively pursue anything until after this surgery. Now that I am past that, I will be more energetic in reinstating my network. I am still hopeful something will work out for me, seeing as how there is a nursing shortage. It is disappointing and discouraging to have that door closed, but there's always a reason why things work out the way they do and I just have to believe that's the case here.

We have daffodils, hyacinths, tulips and irises up in our yard here and it's a gorgeous spring day. We had about three inches of snow on Thursday, but nothing that lasted. I have also seen a couple of butterflies, and the bluebirds are checking out our houses. Tomorrow is March 1 and we'll be hanging out our hummingbird feeders. I'm never ready for it to get too hot, but I enjoy beautiful 65-70 degree days. And even though we all know that celludark looks better than cellulite, I won't be tanning anymore. One experience with chemo is more than enough to last me a lifetime. But I will be outside a lot in the next while--enjoying life and all of the beauty of spring. I'm thankful for the rebirth spring brings, and more thankful I'm here to enjoy it!!

Thank you so very much for all you have meant to us this past year. I can still remember sitting in Dr. Giguere's office for the first time and him asking me, "Where are you parents?" And I had to tell him they were both dead. It was so frightening for me to think it was just going to be Gil and me in this battle, but that turned out to be so wrong!! You have been so constant in your support and we are so humbled by how you have been right beside us this entire year. God certainly knew what He was doing when He gave us friends like you. I know that words cannot express my gratitude adequately, and "thank you" seems so small compared to all you have done for us. I am forever blessed by each of you and I hope you know how much you mean to me. Thank you from the bottom of my heart.

Love,
Susan

THE CANCER RETURNS

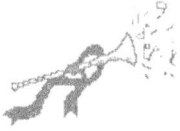

Wednesday, March 30, 2005

Hello to Everyone

I have debated for a while about writing this, but we are so overwhelmed by your calls, e-mails, concern and compassion that I thought it was time to share what's been going on with us so far this year. Gil is not able to keep up with all your questions, and I hate that we can't return all the calls we are receiving, so here goes.

Many of you know I had my "final" breast reconstruction surgery December 28. (The breast implants had not worked out, and I had them removed in July.) This procedure was about 10 hours long, and it brought a large part of my abdomen up to my chest to "create" new breasts. The surgery went well and I came home on New Year's Eve. We were off to a great start in 2005 and I was thankful to have this behind me.

During the surgery, I also had both ovaries removed. My type of breast cancer was off the charts positive for estrogen receptors, and I had been on an anti-cancer medicine for over a year, that supposedly caused my ovaries not to function. Well, it turns out they were working just fine, despite the medication. So we were VERY thankful to have made the decision we did. I saw my oncologist in January for a routine follow up visit and he was delighted with my progress and once again pronounced me cancer free. Which, of course, is the BEST news I can get, anytime!!

However, the healing process hit a bump. Almost immediately after surgery, there were deep purple places on my abdomen that worried the surgeon and us, and it turned out the moving and relocating and re-stretching of tissues caused poor tissue circulation. My incisions began to open by three weeks postop and continued opening until mid-February. We (actually Gil) began packing the wounds and doing dressing changes twice daily in January, in addition to everything he was already doing for me. As the tissue continued to die, I developed black, leathery skin on my abdomen, with dead tissue underneath. This finally progressed to the point that it had to be removed (under anesthesia) in late February. The debridement (removal) left an open wound that was very painful and large. Poor Gil continued to do the packing and dressing changes, and thankfully, we had Home Health nurses coming twice a week to help us.

Gil's parents came and stayed with us for four weeks in late January, just to take some of the burden off Gil. Remember he is self-employed and if he doesn't work, he doesn't make any money. In addition to working, taking care of me, caring for our animals, cooking, shopping, doing laundry, etc., he was "sinking." Based on our experience from all the surgeries of the previous two years, we had planned on my being recovered enough three weeks postop to at least care for myself and be able to stay alone during the day. But I was still almost completely dependent on someone else to help me. We are grateful for his parents being willing to help us out. And yes, his dad even learned to milk goats!!

Well, it's been 13 weeks since surgery and I am progressing slowly. I still have a large wound on my abdomen that requires daily packing and dressing changes. Last week, it was "only" 15 cm x 18 cm large and 1 inch deep. My progress is measured in centimeters, and it will be a while longer before this wound is closed. I also have open wounds on each "breast" that require packing as well. We are hoping to try some new technology speed things along. There is a piece of equipment called a "Wound Vac" that works on the principles of negative pressure/suction to encourage the development of blood supply to the tissue and speed healing. It was placed on me two weeks ago, but was VERY painful and had to be removed. We are scheduled to have it re-applied next week and are hoping for the best. Last week I caught the flu and it set things back a week. I haven't had the flu in many years, and I hope I've had my turn for a while!!! I was very discouraged last week, but through all of this, God continues to have His hand on us, which He shows us daily.

I have been in a recliner since surgery, but am able to get up by myself now, although it is painful and awkward, so if Gil is home, I do ask him "for a hand." Most of the time I have been reading or watching TV, but Gil has a rare day off today and he has helped me get the laptop hooked up and on my lap for a while. I have a small pillow that "lives" on my abdomen for support when changing positions, coughing, etc. and I still have to have Gil help with a shower. He's also still doing all the cooking and housework, but I can get a simple meal together for myself now. So we're "getting there."

We are trying to stay focused on what I can do and how many things we have to be thankful for. One thing we're especially enjoying is spring. Our yard work in the fall is paying off now. We have had crocuses bloom, and are now enjoying daffodils, hyacinths, thrift and forsythia. The tulips are up and the dogwoods in our woods will be opening any day. The bluebirds are checking out the houses and we are awakened every morning with birds singing. We go to sleep at night listening to the baby frogs in the creek and we even heard a "Chuck Will's Widow" call the other night. The weather is perfect right now and we are living with open windows and I'm very thankful for that. I will REALLY be thankful when I can get outside in the yard and get my hands dirty again. One of the benefits of not working and not being able to do much is that I do have 10 perfectly beautiful fingernails for the first time in years!!

In some ways, it's hard to believe spring is here. We have missed a lot so far this year, but we do have so much to be thankful for, and God is good to us. I hope this helps with our communication efforts. Please continue to pray for us--for healing and for grace to endure what God has in store for us. Thank you for your friendship, support, and love.

Susan

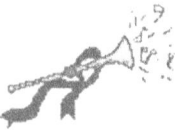

Sunday, December 11, 2005

Hello Everyone

I wanted to ask for your prayers, as God has given us something that seems terrible at this point.

I have been feeling "not good" for about six weeks and when I saw my oncologist on Thursday for a follow up exam, he told my cancer has returned. At this point we are devastated, terrified and just plain numb. We know God doesn't make any mistakes and that His hand is always upon us, but we don't feel very accepting of this situation right now. I keep wanting to tell Him that I've had my turn and been checked off, and that it's not my turn again. But unfortunately, He didn't ask me if I was ready. So we need your prayers.

Please pray for grace for me, because I am so scared right now, I can't think straight. We are at the beginning of a multitude of scans, tests, lab work, needles (my personal favorite) etc. and hopefully we'll know more by the end of the week. I feel so disappointed and let down by this turn of events, even though there were no guarantees given.

Also, please pray that the spread of the cancer is small. I was having specific enough symptoms that they could pinpoint a tumor growing in the bone at the base of my skull and began radiation immediately on Thursday. After only two treatments, there has been improvement in some of the symptoms, and I have at least eight more to go. I still HATE radiation, and now my entire head is engulfed in a mask during the treatment and it freaks me out. It lasts less than five minutes, but it feels like forever. But it does seem to be working. Dr. Giguere did tell me that with the symptoms I was having and with some of the early test results, he wouldn't be surprised if the cancer was growing elsewhere. So please pray specifically that it isn't too widespread.

And third, please pray for Gil. He has been through so much these past two and a half years and is so strong, but this has unnerved him. We both know God doesn't give us anything that He doesn't also give us the ability to handle, but we're at the questioning point still and need to take that leap of faith and trust Him. When we were at the cancer center on Thursday, I saw a poster that said something like, "When we get to the end of the road and life seems to be at its darkest, God either gives us a rock to stand on or wings to fly." We are praying for either right now, and ask that you pray along with us.

I feel selfish for sharing this right before Christmas, but hope that you'll understand and join us in prayer. May God bless each of you as He has always blessed us with YOU.

Love,
Susan

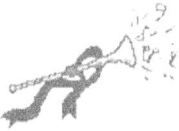

Thursday, December 22, 2005

Hello Everyone.

Greetings from icy Tigerville, SC!!! We had an ice storm that started early Thursday morning and our power has been out since about 8:00 AM Thursday!! Fortunately, in his infinite wisdom, my husband was well-prepared for Y2K and our fireplaces, generator and extra provisions have paid off. We are a little chilly at night, once we turn the generator off for the day, but we really have no complaints. The power company says we should have our power restored by tomorrow, but if not, we are so fortunate to be safe and snug. The phone lines are out as well, so I don't know when this will go out, but hopefully we'll be able to update all of you by Monday. As we were sitting in our warm living room by the fire today, we were reminded about the Hurricane Katrina victims that have been living this way since August, many without a home, and ask you remember them as well.

Well, after a grueling week of tests, scans, needles (remember, my personal favorite?) we have some answers. As always, there is good news and bad news. The good news is that the metastases seem to be only in my bones. I have them in my skull, ribs, spine, hips and femurs (thigh bones). My right hip has been very sore lately and now we know why!! This is the same cancer that grew in my breast two and a half years ago, and one cell just happened to "slip by" chemo and radiation in 2003. Why it's taken this long to set up shop no one knows, but it has started growing with a vengeance.

The PET scan looked like a little "lit up" skeleton--in fact I should be glowing in the dark!! Quite entertaining and interesting, if you're not the patient!! We did ask about the "spots" on my chest X-ray that Dr. Giguere noticed the week before, and he said nothing has shown on any of the scans. He said that doesn't mean the cancer isn't there; just that it may be too early to show up yet. So with his guidance we made our battle plan and have dived into treatment again.

You may remember that my tumor over expressed a gene called Her2Nu. This gene which lives in the cancer cells, causes the cancer cells to produce a protein that in turn cycles back to a receptor on the cancer cells, which stimulates the cancer cells to reproduce. These cancer cells have a nasty little enterprise going, don't they? Back when I was originally diagnosed in 2003, there was a drug in trials called Herceptin. Well, it has passed trials with flying colors and is now available to people like me. I actually started receiving Herceptin on Thursday and will receive it IV on a weekly basis for "I don't know how long" (that's a direct quote from my oncologist). Basically what it does is bind to that receptor on the cancer cells causing two things to happen. First the protein can't bind, so no binding, no growing. However, even more exciting is that it makes the cancer cell have a "red flag" that my immune system recognizes and wants to destroy. So hopefully, it's turning on my immune system to attack the cancer. I am also receiving a drug called Zometa that forces calcium from my blood into my bones. Once the cancer cells are destroyed, it leaves holes, like osteoporosis, and we need calcium in there to rebuild good bone.

The second thing is the radiation and the good it is doing. Remember, I am getting my skull radiated on a daily basis and that I HATE it??? Well, I have had a suggestion that I use that time to pray or meditate. I'm still not calm or happy about it, but I can just about get through the entire 23rd Psalm on one side and the entire Lord's Prayer on the other side of my head before it's over. And the radiation is working. My blistering, blinding headaches have disappeared, the tongue numbness and swallowing difficulties have abated and it's almost like I never had a problem two weeks ago!! I have four treatments left this week on my skull. There is a chance I will also have a few treatments to my right thigh since the mets there are so extensive and it has been so painful for me to go upstairs, get in and out of a car, get in and out of a chair, etc. Gil has been very kind to help pull me to a standing position and our friends and neighbors have been so generous with rides and their time.

And then, when I feel better, (which Dr. Giguere says will be in 2-3 weeks), we're going to start hormone manipulation again with a monthly shot. Remember, my cancer was also estrogen receptor-progesterone receptor positive. So that gives us another angle to attack from. (Remember the part about I hate needles?) Chemo may also be an option further down the road, but nothing either of us wants to discuss yet. Especially me. Dr. Giguere did promise to leave my hair alone this time. It has finally gotten long enough that I had over two inches cut off late in November for the first time. It was so shaggy that it looked bad and just "hung" on my head. So he and I have an understanding about the hair this time. Seriously.

So, even though we've had a very busy week, we feel in much better shape. Dr. Giguere did tell me I was Stage IV, which used to mean terminal, but with all the things they've got going these days, who knows? I've had a very encouraging e-mail from someone who has been Stage IV for 2 and a half years and she's still kicking and fighting. She said I thought I was out of the woods, but I'm not. And I realized I had gotten very complacent about things. It's one thing to know in the back of your head that your disease can come back some day, but another thing altogether to be faced with a "Christmas tree" skeleton on the PET scan and your oncologist telling you that there is no cure for you. He did say he hoped to get things under control and to treat this like a chronic condition, like diabetes. He also said 45 years was not enough time on this planet for anyone!!

I did have three rough days after the Herceptin infusion. For those of you who don't know, the hot flashes of the past two and a half years have been legendary in my house. My poor husband doesn't know whether to wear shorts in winter or a fur coat in July. One of the side effects of Herceptin is either fever or chills.

Well, starting Thursday night, I was feverish from my neck up--red faced, sweating, etc. and under an electric blanket (on 10) from the neck down, literally shaking!! Gil wanted to put my feet to the fireplace and put my head outside in the ice storm!! That was not a fun three days, but it supposedly only is this bad with the first dose. Then my body gets more used to it and it gets better. It was fun to be cold and wear a Christmas sweater for the first time in two years though!!

The other thing I still ask you to pray for is the nausea-thon I've had going on. I managed to lose 15 pounds in a week--and yes that week was just before Christmas thank you very much!! We think the radiation is hitting one or more nausea centers in my brain and that it may be better to suck it up and get it done over the next four days. But I am tired of hauling around a trash can and using it!! It's just not a good look for me!!

Seriously, we thank you all for your prayers, calls, cards, gifts and concern. It has been so good to share with you and lessen our personal burden some. We know God answers prayer and now we just pray that He will use this for His glory.

Merry Christmas!!

Love,
Susan

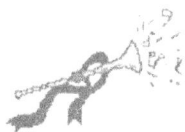

Thursday, January 5, 2006

Hello Everyone and Happy New Year!!

I have had so many of you asking for another update, that I thought it was time to sit down at the computer and write, so here I am.

First of all, we have to thank you for your prayers, encouragement, gifts, meals, phone calls, e-mails and all that you are doing for us. It has been such a blessing to experience the outpouring of support from you, and from people we don't even know who have received our e-mails from you. Thank you for all that you're doing for us, and please continue to pray, because we do believe that God is in control and that He will use this situation. We just aren't sure what we're supposed to do yet, except be faithful.

I have something very exciting to share with you. Remember, I asked you to pray for grace for me? Well, I saw Dr. Giguere on December 21 and of course was asking him a million questions. For example, everything I had read said if the cancer was to return, it would be in the first 18 months. In December I was 32 months out, and was very curious as why now. He said that with the anti-estrogen therapy I had been receiving (tamoxifen and Femara), that the cancer cells had been kept in check, but that eventually they were able to mutate and evolve and develop resistance to these drugs. And when they did, they set up shop and started growing in my bones. Our first line of defense is Herceptin (of which I have now received four doses). I asked him if eventually the cancer would also develop resistance to Herceptin as well, and he said yes. Then he hurried to reassure me that Herceptin was only the first drug in "his arsenal" and he didn't want me to worry because he had lots more options, and research was giving us more options all the time.

Well, I received many e-mails that night, and the one sentence that stuck out in my mind was, "If we truly realized Who walks beside us every day, we would never be afraid." That is so simple, yet so profound to me. As I was drifting off to sleep that night, this sentence was going through my mind. Thursday morning, I don't know if I had a vision, or a dream, or what, but God Himself came and talked to me.

As I was waking up, I could see Dr. Giguere standing in front of me and he was talking about his arsenal and research, etc. and all of a sudden he faded away and I could feel God's presence right in front of my face. And He said, "I've got this. I've always had this, but you need to let it go and give it to Me." Remember that I said I was walking around with an icy fear inside me? It was almost like He was saying to me, I've given you two weeks to be afraid, angry, upset, etc., but now it's time to give it to Me. Well, when I realized this was God talking to me, I started to cry and tell Him how sorry I was. Then I did give Him all of it. And I had such a sense of peace. When I began to thank Him, He then gave me joy. And then I woke all the way up. Of course, I had to wake up Gil and tell him. And it was the most wonderful gift I've ever been given. What a Christmas present to receive.

I had to go to the cancer center later that morning for my last dose of radiation and Dr. Giguere saw me in the waiting room and asked me if I was okay. I said yes, and he told me I looked different. I was able to tell him that God had spoken to me that morning and after he left, the other patients in the waiting room wanted to hear my story. So I told them and we had a praise session right there. We all realized that God is bigger than any cancer any of us had and that He was, and is, in control. People were even telling me my face looked different. So often we pray and ask God for His presence, but when it does happen, it is so unbelievable that you almost don't realize what happened till it's over. He did take me to a new level with Him, and I was able to truly realize Who was walking beside me. And He has given me grace to withstand whatever this new chapter brings to us. Usually, I am one to give my troubles to God, but then five minutes later, I want to tell Him how to handle what I've just given Him. This time is different, and I haven't had one moment of fear or doubt since that morning.

And what an awesome start to our Christmas weekend. We were able to make the 11:00 PM Christmas Eve service that we always go to and it was absolutely wonderful. I started going to the late service with my friend Mary in high school, and I don't think we've missed a service since. Christmas Day was very quiet for us--we had a fire in the fireplace and just watched movies and enjoyed each other. Gil made a beautiful Christmas dinner (with a little help from me) and we had a GREAT day.

So I have now received a total of four doses of Herceptin, the most recent being yesterday. I am starting to feel better, but have no stamina to speak of. My appetite has returned and the nausea-thon is over -- hallelujah!!! I see Dr. Giguere next Thursday and get lab work done. I am eager and anxious to see how the lab work looks. My red blood cell count was so low the last time I saw him that I have been receiving a shot (yes more needles) called Aranesp every other week that is supposed to stimulate the production of RBCs. My white cells were low enough that he told me to stay away from sick people, little kids, crowds, etc. and I have been very good in that regard. I just don't have a lot of extra energy right now, but I am getting time to cross stitch, read, etc.

So that's where we are. I hope each of you had wonderful Christmas and New Year's holidays with your families. We are so blessed to have so many wonderful people in our lives who care about us and want what is best for us. We are truly thankful for each of you and wish you a very Happy 2006.

Love,
Susan

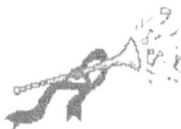

Monday, February 27, 2006

Hello Everyone.

I know many of you have been wondering what's going on in our world. I saw the oncologist on Feb. 15 and we've had a couple of challenging weeks. We appreciate all your phone calls and support, and have been truly overwhelmed by your compassion. Since it has been a couple of weeks, I'll go chronologically with this update. There has been a lot going on, and I'll try to make it as organized as possible.

Remember me saying I don't like seeing Dr. Giguere right now because every time I do, he tells me something else I don't want to hear? This visit was no exception. We started out by discovering my hemoglobin had continued to drop. For those of you non-medical folks, this is a measure of red blood cells and the normal range is 12-16. Mine was 10.4 in December, 9.7 in January and 8.2 at this visit. I have been taking iron pills daily and receiving a shot (that hurts like h___) every other week to help stimulate the production of red blood cells. Obviously, this wasn't working well enough, and 8.2 is a dangerous level. What was odd was that all my other blood counts remained about where they were previously. So I had to have a transfusion of two units of packed red cells the following day at the hospital. The nursing staff was wonderful and took great care of me. Blood has to run in slowly, so I was there for about five hours--a very long day for me. When I got home, I was feeling a little queasy, but chalked that up to being tired.

We didn't have my tumor marker available on Wednesday since it takes longer to run than "regular" lab work and I was too tired to worry about it on Thursday. I still wasn't feeling good--kind of nauseated and tired, but thought it must be nerves. Well, Friday Dr. Giguere called me with more bad news. The marker, which was 297 in December and 293 in January had risen to 577--almost doubling itself. This meant the Herceptin wasn't stopping the spread of the cancer and that there was more of it growing inside me.

Dr. Giguere wanted me to start chemo Monday--and you have to know I wasn't happy about that. The poor man answered a million questions and was very patient with me, but I still wasn't pleased. The chemo drug is called Xeloda and you take it in pill form. It is absorbed in one form through the digestive tract, and then an enzyme in the blood converts it to its active form. It supposedly "finds" Herceptin and potentiates it. This means that if Herceptin is 2 and Xeloda is 2, that $2 + 2$ equals 7 inside the body. Dr. Giguere also said most people don't get sick and there is no hair loss.

By about 7:00 PM Friday night, I was really feeling bad and started vomiting. I couldn't keep anything in my stomach all weekend. Gil called the cancer center on Monday and told them I was sick and they had him pick up some phenergan--an anti-nausea drug. This helped the nausea fade a little, but it never went away. When I finally went for my regularly scheduled appt. at the cancer center on Wednesday, I was still vomiting and had lost 15 lbs. I didn't get any herceptin that day, but did receive two liters of fluid, along with a cocktail of anti-nausea medicine, sedatives and steroids. Again, this ran in over almost five hours, so I was really tired. And since I couldn't swallow anything for almost a week, I hadn't had any ibuprofen and my bone pain was really making itself known.

There was talk of IV chemo if I couldn't take the pills because we have to get the cancer in check. However, I managed to eat half a plain baked potato on Wednesday night and keep it down!!! Thursday morning I ate a piece of toast

80

which also stayed down, and had to go back to the cancer center for more fluids and herceptin. We were all thrilled that I was feeling better and I managed to start taking the Xeloda Thursday night. I have to eat a meal, wait an hour and then take four pink pills--not without a little trepidation, and drink a big glass of water. This has to be done twice daily, and so far so good. I have felt a little nauseous in the mornings because I'm not used to eating so much food so early, but that's been the worst of it.

The chemo is a fourteen day round, and then I get a week off (for good behavior??). Then we measure my tumor marker and if it is down, we start again. Dr. Giguere said his goal is to have the number in double digits SOON!! So I am eating okay now--still nothing too heavy. I know it's probably in my mind, but I am taking chemo and don't want to be sick like before.

The other GREAT news is that my abdominal wound has FINALLY closed-- after fourteen months. I still have two small tunnels that have to be packed and dressed twice daily, but the big wound is healed!!! It was initially over 10 inches across--hard to imagine, but now it is closed over!!!!

On a beautiful note, we know God still has His hand on this--I had to tell myself that very frequently in the last two weeks. But now that I feel better, He has shown me the beginning of His glorious spring. We have cheerful yellow daffodils and beautiful yellow and purple crocuses beginning to bloom in our yard--along with lavender thrift. I haven't been able to do any yard work in the past year, so this is "leftovers" from our previous years' work.

We also had a pair of bluebirds "checking out" one of our houses this morning and a Carolina wren singing his heart out. It's just wonderful to watch the rebirth of God's world for another year. It is so good to know that no matter where we are, He remains constant in our lives. And we can always count on Him--just like the coming of spring and the renewal of life.

Thank you all for your prayers. We are so grateful to have your support. I hope you enjoy the gift of today!!

Love,
Susan

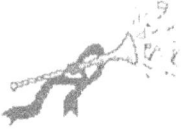

Monday, March 20, 2006

Hello Everyone.

Well, it's been another four weeks since our last update and we have wonderful news to share with you this time!!!! We know God answers prayers, but not always with the answer we have been wanting to hear. We also know that you have been praying for us and that you have asked your families and friends to pray as well. We receive mail from folks we don't even know who let us know they are remembering us to our Father, and it is so humbling to realize so many people care about us. Thank you, thank you, thank you for your prayers and support.

Well, onto the "report." I was at the cancer center on Wednesday for my weekly visit. I got lab work done and once again my hemoglobin had dropped significantly to 8.8 (normal is 12-16). Dr. Giguere said he had to take off his oncology hat and put on his hematology hat to try to figure out what is going on, because all my other numbers are staying about the same. The other blood counts are still low, but not dropping off like the hemoglobin. He thinks the anemia is unrelated to the cancer or the chemo, and that something else is going on. Meanwhile, I needed blood, so I spent five hours at the hospital yesterday receiving a transfusion. Special thanks to Janet, who brought me lunch and made the afternoon fly by with her visit.

After I left the hospital, I called home the check messages and Dr. Giguere's nurse practitioner had called and left a message for me. You may remember that my tumor marker has been rising since December and that it was 577 in February. I started taking an oral chemo right after that. Well, the wonderful news is that my tumor marker had dropped to 274 on Wednesday--less than half of what it was!!! So the chemo is working to kill the cancer cells!!!! The drug is called Xeloda and is not without side effects, but I feel like I've been given the spoonful of sugar to get the medicine down!! I have to eat a meal, then take four pills and drink a big glass of water twice a day. I am very full, bloated and queasy for about an hour afterwards, but knowing what we do now, I'll trade two hours of queasy for success!! I take the pills for 14 days, and then I get a week off. I lost 10 lbs. while taking the chemo, but managed to gain five back last week (my "off" week)!! It also makes me VERY tired, so I don't have much energy. But that's a small trade off as well!! I started taking the drug again yesterday and will finish this round March 29. Then I'll get another week off and see Dr. Giguere before starting back again. He really thinks that the tumor marker number will be into double digits soon.

With my hemoglobin dropping so much, I have been taking a horse pill of iron every night as well. But Dr. Giguere has also decided that we need to go to IV iron because apparently I am not absorbing what I'm eating. So beginning next week, my days at the cancer center will be 8+ hours long. I will get a test dose of iron (it can cause a severe systemic reaction), then we have to wait an hour, then I get loaded up on Benadryl (to mediate any potential reaction), then I get herceptin, then the iron infuses over a minimum of 6 hours. And I'm told that you can develop a reaction to IV iron over time, so this is the protocol every week. Fortunately, I have lots of books, puzzles, cross stitch, etc. to occupy my time when I'm not sleeping off the Benadryl!!

I also wanted to share another experience with you. I have been learning that even when our days seem darkest, we always have something to thankful for. Sometimes it's just the fact that we wake up and have the gift of a new day. Instead of focusing on what's going on in my body, I have been trying to focus on praising God. And there is an old song that I love that says:

Praise the Lord; He can work through those who praise Him

Praise the Lord, for our God inhabits praise.

Praise the Lord, and the chains that seem to bind you, fall powerless behind you when you praise Him.

I haven't been able to get that song out of my head for a couple of weeks now. It's easy to see God in our beautiful spring weather and all the flowers and trees that are blooming right now. But on cold, dark days, sometimes we have to look a little harder. Since December, I haven't liked what I've been hearing from Dr. Giguere. But I decided that I would praise God no matter what. And He has shown me that He does inhabit our praise. What a great thing to learn!!! Thank you for letting me share this with you and for all your prayers, cards, calls, e-mails and all the other ways you support us. We love each of you and are so thankful for you. May God bless you as you praise him!! Have a GREAT weekend!!

Love,
Susan

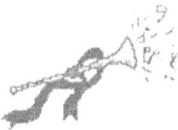

Friday, April 7, 2006

Hello Everyone.

It's been three weeks since my last update, and this time we've had good news and great news!! So it's time to share.

I saw the oncologist on Wednesday, and my hemoglobin had actually climbed to 11.3!!! This is the highest it has been (without transfusions) since we learned of about the return of my cancer in early December. The week prior it had been 10.6, so this number is heading in the right direction. And since the number was so good, I didn't have to do the iron marathon on Wednesday. An extra hug and thank you to Brenda, who has been such a special friend to stay with me ALL DAY LONG on those 8+ hour days and also to Hope, for a wonderful visit AND lunch last week.

Being a nurse has its benefits, and the previous week, the cancer center nurses and I worked it out so I could be at the cancer center at 8:00 on Wednesday, and they would go ahead and give me everything except iron before I saw Dr. Giguere. By the time I saw him, it was almost 10:00 and he ordered one more drug that infused over 20 minutes. So I was out of there by 11:00 (and I can tell you the door did not hit me in the rear end on my way out). For those of you who don't live in our beautiful corner of the world, it was such a gift to have the afternoon free. Our spring is in full bloom--literally and it was sunny, with low humidity and about 80 degrees. I was so thankful for that time to just enjoy our weather and flowers and birds and butterflies. We had our first hummingbird show up at the feeder on Tuesday, so spring has officially arrived!!

And as if that weren't enough good news, I got a phone call on Thursday about my tumor marker. Remember last time it had plummeted from 577 to 274? This time, the number was 167. Which means, the nasty, I mean wonderful, pink pills (chemo) are working. I started my third round yesterday morning and was grumbling about having to take them again, and how it was only one out of 28 times, etc. After that phone call, the pills went down much easier last night. (I guess you could say the call was the spoonful of sugar!!) The only downside was that I was hit with pretty significant fatigue yesterday. I guess I felt so good on my week off, I "forgot" what it is to take chemo!! However, with this kind of news, I won't complain about feeling tired. And Dr. Giguere told me he wanted to have this number in the double digits soon, so now the race is on.

Between screaming with delight and shedding tears of joy yesterday afternoon, I realized the 167 was like God had placed a giant billboard right in front of me to remind me, yet again, that all of this is part of His plan. Since my special time with Him before Christmas, I haven't been afraid of anything, but some days are really challenging. Yesterday was such a vivid reminder of His love for us.

And on Wednesday, when I was driving into the cancer center, I was having a wonderful pity party for myself. I never want to go in there, but this week my attitude was especially bad. I was really busy thinking about how unfair this was, etc. and I turned on the radio for distraction. The announcer came on and was sharing about a bible passage he had read earlier that morning. It talked about (paraphrasing) how He who was without sin became sin, so we could become righteous. Talk about not fair!! Once again, God in His gentle way threw a brick right at me and made His point. What a great message the week before Easter.

I want thank all of you for all the cards, calls, encouragement, but mostly your prayers. Please continue to pray for us and that God will give us the courage to graciously endure what He has planned for us. Thank you for your love and friendship. May God bless each of you and Happy Easter!!!

Love,
Susan

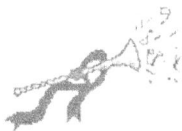

Monday, June 5, 2006

Hello Everyone

I know it's been a while since I've sent out an update, and I appreciate all the calls, e-mails, cards and especially the prayers from you. I have been very tired and not feeling well for a while, and I do apologize for not feeling talkative lately. But here's what's been going on, and I hope you'll understand.

Four weeks ago we had bad news, in that my tumor marker had gone from 163 to 274. Dr. Giguere wasn't concerned and told me to continue with the oral chemo (Xeloda) and Herceptin infusion. So now four more weeks have passed and the tumor marker rose from 274 to 446.

I had my monthly office visit with Dr. Giguere on Wednesday of last week and he kept telling me how good I looked. When he asked how I was feeling I told him okay but that the fatigue was really getting to me. It's awful to wake up exhausted, and then have to take pills that make you more tired!! We discussed alternatives to the Xeloda, but he said he didn't want to do anything until we had my tumor marker results. So now I have "failed" the Herceptin/Xeloda combination twice, and it's time to progress to intravenous chemo. Dr. Giguere said his goals were to keep me medically safe and clinically intact. (He told me my hair looked beautiful on Wednesday, and I told him he was not allowed to discuss, touch, or even think about my hair, so obviously my goals are in reverse order from his!! Ha Ha). I don't remember the name of the new drug, but I get it IV once a week for two weeks, and then have a week off.

I will continue to get the Herceptin weekly for now. The new drug is a cousin of Taxol (which I had in the first rounds of chemo three years ago) and I did okay on that. Of course, my main concern is the nausea and vomiting routine that has become so familiar to me and I DON'T intend to go through that again.

On the upside, I will just have to deal with drugs once a week instead of twice daily for two weeks. Even if I have a crummy day or two, it's better than two weeks of the "yucks" and having to eat and feel bloated and queasy just so I can take poison.

I still believe God is guiding this journey for us, and even though I don't understand exactly what His plan is, I am not afraid or worried about what's going to happen. I have had a few moments of sadness because I love life here on earth, but I saw a church billboard this weekend that said "Turn your eyes upon Jesus and look full in His wonderful face." As you already know, the rest of the verse says, "and the things of earth will grow strangely dim in the light of His glory and grace." So maybe I just need to re-focus my "lens" and priorities.

When Dr. Giguere talked to me on Thursday, he told me we would start the IV chemo on June 14. He wanted to give my body a break and told me he was not concerned and that I should just get out have a great time for the next little while. Of course, I was ready to go back into the cancer center and start the chemo on Friday, but he said no. So we had a cold front come through on Friday, and Saturday was the perfect day. Sunny, Carolina blue skies, a light breeze and about 80 degrees. So we got in the car and had a road trip. We drove to Caesar's Head in N. Greenville County and the sky was so clear you could see to Georgia!! We have never been there when it wasn't cloudy, humid, foggy or something. Needless to say, my shutterbug husband went nuts taking pictures. Then we drove to Brevard and on up to the Blue Ridge Parkway. The mountain laurel was in full bloom and the rhododendrons were getting started. The perfect weather continued, and we even had a picnic on the grass at one of the overlooks. We drove all the way to Mt. Mitchell (the highest peak in the Eastern US) but it was too chilly to do much outside!! The temp was 54 degrees and the winds were gusting to 20 mph, making it feel like 40 degrees. In June!!! It was absolutely beautiful to be "on top of the world" with the vistas that go on forever. We drove home the long way and were VERY tired, but relaxed. We had the dogs with us and Sadie has to always be looking out the window or standing on the divider between the front seats, supervising. Needless to say, she has been in a coma since we got home Saturday evening. Yesterday was a rest day for me, and today I feel better. I do have more energy when I'm not taking chemo and it feels good!!

I have even been working in the yard a little. Of course, Gil has done most of the work, but we have our garden in and everything has sprouted. He planted tomatoes, corn, sunflowers, okra, gourds, pumpkins, beans, peas, cucumbers, peppers, herbs and zucchini. We had two neighbors bring goodies from their gardens yesterday, so we are looking forward to sharing ours when it matures. We also planted annuals in the flower beds and they look so pretty.

It's been three years since I've been able to work in the yard, and Gil has been a good sport about crawling around on the ground so I can have something pretty to look at. And we've had tons of butterflies on the new plants already. And if that weren't enough, we're enjoying hummingbird wars at our feeders. We have seen one female and three males for sure--there may be more, but the feeder is apparently the "in" place for hummers in our neighborhood.

Also, my brother David was here for a visit three weeks ago. He lives in Houston and wanted to get away from the heat for a while. We didn't do a whole lot, but we did get a chance to catch up. I haven't seen him in almost three years, so it was nice to have him here for a visit.

So that's where we are. Thank you again for your concern and caring, but most especially for your prayers. I hope you are enjoying the start of a beautiful summer and that you will be richly blessed, as we all are with you.

Love,
Susan

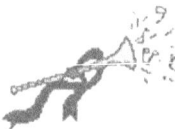

Thursday, July 27, 2006

Greetings from HOT and sunny South Carolina, where it's summertime and the livin' is easy. Well, sort of.

We did have good news yesterday. When I last wrote, it was just before starting intravenous chemo. The good news is that this seems to be working better than oral chemo. The great news is that my tumor marker has gone from the high 400s in early June, to 141 yesterday. This is the lowest it has been since we were hit by the bulldozer in December. I am trying not to get too excited, because it has come down before, only to go higher the next time. The bad news is that I have not had good counts and am continuing to receive "booster" shots for low red blood cells and white blood cells. Dr. Giguere says this is because the chemo is working at the level of the bone marrow and that along with killing the cancer cells, it is also "messing with" my good blood cells.

The chemo I'm getting is called Abraxane and it infuses over a half hour, once a week for three weeks, then I get a week off. I am still getting Herceptin because apparently in the oncology world, if Abraxane is 2 and Herceptin is 1, then $2 + 1 = 5$ when they are given together. I also get a steroid called Decadron (I guess I won't be trying out for any sports teams this fall) and a drug called Zometa once a month (which is supposed to take calcium out of my blood and put it into my bones). With the cancer growing there, there is an increased risk of pathological fractures.

More good news. I had a PET scan in late June, which showed "remarkable resolution of soft tissue involvement," which in English says there is no cancer in any of my organs--just my bones. There were some lymph nodes in my neck and some lung masses that showed up in December, but they are now gone. So I had to go for another bone scan, and it "was a little worse" which in English meant there were "a couple of new lesions showing up in my skull." The other areas (ribs, hips, spine and femurs) were either no worse or better than the scan in December. So the good news is that the cancer is confined to my bones for now. I still hurt all the time and take ibuprofen around the clock, but am much more mobile and flexible than earlier in the year.

The horrible news is that while the Abraxane is working on my cancer, it has also taken most of my hair again. You may remember that was my biggest trauma last time, and it has been an adjustment again. I cried for several weeks, and still feel like I'm looking at a stranger in the mirror, but I guess this is a small sacrifice in exchange for life. I heard from another chemo patient who had just lost his hair, that he focused on the Bible verse that says God even knows the number of hairs on our head. He said this just made it easier on God to keep track of his. So in the face of this loss, we can still laugh. I still have enough hair to get away with wearing a baseball cap for now--I have several fashion colors!! But I have purchased another wig for when I will need to wear one again.

I also have an area of numbness in my left jaw that has been present for this whole year. Sometimes it is completely numb, and others it tingles and is painful. Imagine someone holding an ice cube to your lower jaw and that is close to what it feels like. Well, now a mass has "appeared" on my jawbone in the form of a bump that can be felt, so I see the radiation oncologist again next week. I'll probably have to get another "hockey mask" made and have focal radiation to that one area. You know how I detest radiation and having my head bolted to the bed, but if it will make this better, then I'm ready for it.

Meanwhile, our garden is flourishing--we are picking handfuls of cherry tomatoes almost every day and eating them like candy. We've also had lots of zucchini, peppers, green beans, big tomatoes and herbs. The corn is tasseling and our sunflowers are about 8 feet tall and blooming, and soon we'll be eating okra. Gil also picked his first two cucumbers this week and they are good!! We've also had wonderful neighbors sharing blueberries, squash and corn, so we are well fed with this season's bounty. I do not thrive in the heat and humidity (I count the days till September, when cooler, drier weather is the norm) so it's wonderful to look outside and see life flourishing in the summer.

We are also quite entertained with the hummingbird wars going on at our feeders from before sunrise till dark. We always get excited when the first one shows up in March, but when there are 8 or more at a time, doing their aerial acrobatics, it is really fun to watch. I am filling feeders every other day, which is a fun chore.

We're also doing some redecorating of our upstairs. Gil moved into a new office in June and decided to take his big desk, several bookcases, and other furniture from his home office to his new office. So we've moved the guest bedroom into his old office, where there is much more room. Of course, once that room got emptied out, we had to paint and wallpaper it, clean the carpet, etc. Well, that has escalated into every room needing a wallpaper border or something, all the closets needing to be cleaned out, etc. So we are in the middle of this project. The good news is that it does look nice when we're finished, and we will have more room for our guests.

Well, that's about it for now. We thank you so much for your continued support of us with your prayers, calls, cards and all the other ways you show you care. May God bless each of you.

Love,
Susan

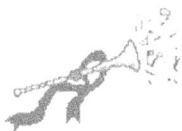

Wednesday, September 6, 2006

Hello Everyone,

It's been a while since our last update, and I do appreciate your calls, cards, offers of meals and other support. I've had a very rough three weeks and I'm sorry I haven't been more available. One of the schedulers at the Cancer Center has the following taped to her computer and I've really needed to hear it:

"When you get to the end of all the light you know and it's time to step into the darkness of the unknown, faith is knowing that one of two things shall happen: Either you will be given something solid to stand on, or you will be taught how to fly."

I love reading that and believe me there has been a lot of living in faith these past few weeks.

You may remember that I was to receive 10 doses of radiation for an area on my left lower jaw. Except for some nausea and vomiting (more motion sickness than anything), that went smoothly. I did have my head bolted to the bed during the treatments and I still hate radiation, but the "bump" on my jaw is gone and the numbness has almost totally resolved. That's the good news. Dr. Wilcox told me I may get a burned area in my mouth, but what she didn't tell me was that almost my whole mouth (including my tongue) would be blistered. That started the last day of radiation and is still getting better. For almost two weeks, I could only eat tiny bites on the back right side of my mouth and it had to be room temperature, very soft food. Along with that, I seemed to be on the nausea/vomiting/diarrhea diet and have lost 13 pounds in the last two weeks. I know you are jealous, but this is not the way to do it!!! However, that seems to be getting better too. My stomach is still sensitive, but I am eating more and the blisters are almost gone. I don't care how much cancer is in my jaw, I'm not sure I want to do that again!! The good part of the radiation is that we also radiated my lower spine. That has hurt since December and Dr. Wilcox reviewed my bone scans with me. There was significant spread of the cancer from December 2005 till June 2006 in that area. As soon as the radiation was finished there, there was no more pain and I have been pain free in my back since.

I also continued chemo during this time, and with the double whammy, the yucky days were worse. However, I did have a week off from chemo last week. I still didn't feel good, but at least I wasn't adding insult to injury. We did get to the Apple Festival in Hendersonville, NC last Saturday and it was a cool, rain free day. I was very short of breath and had to stop and rest every two blocks or so, but we had a good time and it was absolutely charming. Gil was very patient with me and bought me a beautiful scarecrow. (He got to eat apple funnel cakes, so he wasn't too deprived.) It was a very nice outing, but I paid for it the rest of the weekend.

I saw Dr. Giguere yesterday and we had a long talk. My hemoglobin had dropped to 9 (normal is 12-16) so he started me on oral iron in addition to the IV medication. But that's a wonderful explanation as to why I am so tired and short of breath. What I haven't told you is that two weeks ago, my tumor marker was up to 230 from 141. As badly as I have been feeling, I was very discouraged. But he said it's not time to be worried yet. Since it went from 362 to 141 previously, the 141 may have been a "false low" because that was such a huge drop, and the 230 may be a more accurate reading. I'm still not dancing on the ceiling, but he did tell me this would be my last cycle of Abraxane. So with the treatment I got yesterday, I have two more weeks and then I'm done with that. Of course I had to ask him what was next, but he said he didn't know yet. But he did think it was time for my body to have a break, since we've been beating it up this whole year. He's even considering taking me off herceptin and trying another growth inhibitor for at least a month just to have time for me to recover. He told me it was time for some r and r and r. (Rest, recreation and regrowth of hair!!) Of course, I'll get another tumor marker measurement in two weeks and that will be the real determining factor. But 4 cycles of Abraxane is about the maximum anyone gets, and I'm maxed out!!! So please continue to pray for us, to be faithful no matter what God has in store for us. It's scary to be at this spot of uncertainty without a roadmap. But I guess that's exactly what faith is!!

On a much happier note, it's after Labor Day here and we're eagerly anticipating fall. Cooler temperatures, lower humidity, turning leaves, pumpkins, and all the beauty of the season. Plus college football games--go 'noles!! Gil got out all of our scarecrows, pumpkins, leaves, etc. for inside the house and I must say, he did a wonderful job. So even though the trees outside are still green, we can be excited what's to come. Fall is my very favorite time of year and I can't wait for open windows, fires in the fireplace, a pot of chili or soup simmering on the stove, and sleeping under a warm electric blanket again. We have picked about 2 dozen mini pumpkins and gourds from the garden, and Gil has saved his cornstalks for me. Our giant sunflowers are about ready to harvest, and we had neighbors bring over apples from the trees!! You can almost feel the snap in the air. The only sad thing about summer ending is that "our" hummingbirds will soon be migrating south. We are still enjoying their "wars" at the feeders and won't take them in till the end of the month.

Thanks for letting me share my ups and downs with you. We do appreciate your prayers and continue to pray for you. May God bless you as He continues to bless us with your friendship and love.

Love,
Susan

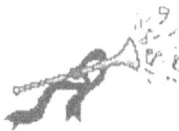

Thursday, November 9, 2006

Hello Everyone.

What a challenging time we have had recently. We appreciate being in your prayers because that's the only thing that has gotten us through the last four weeks. We've had many calls and offers of support and we do appreciate all your kindnesses, but the best thing anyone can do now is to pray for us.

At the end of September, I got my last dose of Abraxane (chemo) and was going to be in a study for a new experimental drug called Tykerb. It is not chemo, but blocks the Her2nu gene in more ways than Herceptin. It is not approved by the FDA yet, so by participating in the clinical trials I essentially agreed to be a guinea pig. Because it isn't considered chemo, it is not as hard on my body and theoretically I would get a break from all the chemo (poisons) they have been giving me. So we decided to take a mini-vacation to celebrate. We had some of our best friends invite us to Litchfield Beach to stay with them and were able to go the last weekend in September. It was not crowded, we had perfect weather and even saw dolphins past the breakers.

When we returned home, the following week, I started with the nausea/vomiting routine and was very dizzy. I spent the better part of two days at my old hospital, getting a bone scan, CT scan, X-rays, an EKG, and an MRI of my brain. Special thanks to Amanda in pre-op for starting two great IVs for me. (I am a horrible stick, and usually I end up feeling like a pin cushion). These were all in preparation for starting the new drug. The clinical trials required baseline scans, then periodic scans throughout the trial. On Friday, after finishing up at the hospital, I went to the cancer center to have blood drawn for lab work. I mentioned that I had been dizzy and vomiting for three days and couldn't keep anything down and wanted to see the doctor or the nurse practitioner.

What I didn't know was that the radiologist from the hospital had already read all my scans and called with bad news. So when I saw the nurse practitioner, she told me that my cancer had metastasized to my brain. She said I had two tumors that showed on the MRI and that I needed to start radiation immediately. Thankfully, Gil was with me because this freaked me out. She said that my oncologist was out of town, and would see me Tuesday. As it turned out I saw my oncologist, and the radiation oncologist, then got a new form of chemo called Gemzar that Tuesday. They also gave me some powerful anti-nausea medication along with steroids. Apparently the nausea and dizziness was coming from where the cancer was growing in my brain because there is no room inside your cranium, so anything "extra" like a tumor causes symptoms. Dr. Wilcox (the radiation oncologist) told us that brain tissue is very resistant to radiation while cancer is very vulnerable to radiation so that was the perfect route. She also told me I had six visible tumors on the MRI and showed them to us. And since I had six visible tumors, I probably had dozens more "seeds" so the plan was to radiate my entire brain, even though the visible tumors were only in one area.

So I started radiation to my brain (remember how I love having my head bolted to the table and that machine circling around and making all kinds of funky noise?) on Wednesday. Dr. Giguere (my oncologist) didn't want to give me any chemo during radiation because that would be too much for my body to handle. Meanwhile, before that first dose of Gemzar the day before radiation, my tumor marker had climbed to 690. Another reason to freak out, since that is the highest it has ever been. After two weeks, the radiation was complete and the dizziness and most of the nausea was gone, thank goodness. I got another dose of Gemzar on Tuesday of last week, and was still exhausted and sleeping a lot. This week, my blood counts were too low to get chemo, but the good news is that with the two doses of Gemzar, my tumor marker was down to 527. Still way too high for my comfort level, but at least it was down significantly. I also had a flu shot and Gil is getting his Friday. My white blood cells are dangerously low right now, but without chemo this week, hopefully they will bounce back up.

Since I "failed" my scans and because you can't have any other treatment going on at the same time you are taking Tykerb, I am not eligible for the clinical trials. However, when I saw Dr Giguere this past Tuesday, he said they are doing all the paperwork to get me in this study as a "compassionate patient," meaning I'll still get the drug, while receiving chemo. His plan is for me to have Gemzar and herceptin every other week, and then take Tykerb during the "off" weeks. I don't know where this will take us in this ongoing battle, but we have faith and know this is part of God's plan.

Meanwhile, I have lost just about all my hair and can't get away with just a baseball cap anymore. It has turned into a beautiful fall, and I only have one complaint. My ears are cold!! We have wonderful well water at our house and we have been telling folks how good it is, but looking and Gil and me, you might want to reconsider before you drink it!!

We did have some very special visitors two weekends ago. My next door neighbors growing up in Florida who were like parents to me, took a road trip from Florida and visited friends in Georgia, North Carolina and us. They were able to stay the whole weekend, and we drove the mountain roads looking at the gorgeous leaves in N. Greenville County and N. Carolina (God's country) one day, then went to downtown Greenville, Furman, and the local sites another day. The weather was perfect and we had a great time. Gil took 2 days off work and was the perfect host. Since I get tired so easily, he really pitched in and did a great job with meals, driving, building fires in the fireplace and everything else. It was tiring for me, but I wouldn't trade their visit for anything. They are so special to both of us, and it was a real pleasure having them. And "our" deer even put in an appearance one morning. First we saw one doe with one fawn, and then we saw another doe with two fawns. What a treat!!

Meanwhile, fall continues to be absolutely glorious here. In Greenville the trees are just now getting their full colors and you can't go anywhere without appreciating their beauty. We have been quite cool (our first frost was Oct. 13), but today is supposed to be 75 degrees and sunny. I guess we'll get a dose of Indian summer. I had asked God earlier in the year to please let me live long enough to see fall. He has done that, and now I find I'm greedy and want to make it to Christmas. I guess we humans always want more.

So that's our update for now. Please continue to pray for us that we'll have the courage to accept what God has planned for us. We haven't liked His plan much lately, but I realize that the valleys are as important as the mountaintops. Thank you for all the ways you encourage us. May God give you a special blessing today.

Love,
Susan

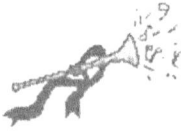

Saturday, December 23, 2006

Hello Everyone,

Gil and I met with Dr. Giguere this week and it wasn't exactly what we wanted to hear, but at least we are dealing with the truth. I truly have not felt good since the end of September and wanted something more that another prescription for pain, nausea, etc. I wasn't supposed to see anyone for an office visit, just get my infusion, and have a break from chemo this week. But I have been so nauseated and in pain that I called on Tuesday and told the nurse I wanted to talk to Dr. Giguere when I was there on Wednesday. Well, she waved her magic wand and got me in to see him that next morning.

Gil was able to come with me and ask questions too, and we are thankful for that. I basically told Dr. Giguere that I had been feeling like crap (yes, that was the word I used) for three months and wanted to know what was going on inside my body. He told me that my underlying disease (he refuses to say cancer) was causing some of the problems but he was convinced that the treatment was responsible for some of the symptoms as well. I told him I was tired of hurting all the time and being nauseated or sick all the time too. (I lost another 10-1/2 lbs. last week.) The latest is I can only eat about 3-4 bites, and it feels like the food is at the top of my esophagus at the back of my throat for hours. It just won't go down. So I asked him about that and told him all I could eat was applesauce or maybe half a banana and that's only about twice a day. He said he didn't have an answer for that but ordered another PET scan (which I will have next Friday). You may remember that looks at all the organs for possible involvement and takes about 2 hours in Nuclear Medicine.

We talked about my tumor marker continuing to rise, despite chemo and I told him I felt like this indicated chemo wasn't working and he said basically, yes, that was right. Yet part of my nausea and vomiting is from the chemo. So he said that perhaps we should stop chemo for now and Gil and I agreed that we should. This is a very scary step for us because it means there is nothing that I am taking now that will kill the cancer cells. We did agree to hormone therapy, which will slow/stop the replication of the cancer cells but it doesn't kill what's already there. I had two shots of a new drug called Faslodex that is an anti-hormonal before I left the cancer center on Wednesday and I should receive those monthly until . . .

We are also trying to get me involved with the experimental drug Tykerb, but that could take till March. So we've set out on uncharted territory and are really in need of your prayers. I don't know what will happen without chemo. If this is God's timing and I am to go Home soon, please pray that I will be strong in Him and able to do what He asks. If this is not His time yet, please pray that I feel better, because I have been feeling really crummy for about three months, have lost too much weight (there's the irony in all this--me who has struggled with her weight all her life, is almost too thin now!!) and am not able to do much of anything for myself anymore.
God has been with us through this and we know He continues to have His hand on all we do, but it is sometimes difficult not to question Him.

We are certain He has blessed us with each of you and your continued love, support and friendship. Special thanks to Pam, Lisa, Brenda, and Roxie for rides to/from the cancer center. I am not driving right now so am dependent on the kindness of our friends and it has been unwavering as always. Please continue to pray for us as we continue to thank God for each of you. Merry Christmas and may we all remember what CHRISTmas is truly about.

Love,
Susan

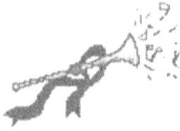

Thursday, January 11, 2007

Hello Everyone.

Thank you for being a friend and prayer partner through Susan's journey with cancer. This past weekend, things took a turn for the worse and Susan is now in the Critical Care Unit of St. Francis Hospital (downtown). She asked me to write this message on her behalf because she cannot do it herself.

On Saturday she began to complain of breathing difficulties and shortness of breath. As the day progressed it got worse and her doctors ultimately told her to go to the emergency room. They initially suspected a blood clot in her lungs but it ultimately proved to be a heavy concentration of what appears to be cancerous fluids between her lungs and the rib cage (tests are not back yet). They removed about 750cc of fluid (almost a quart) and she began breathing easier.

On Monday she was scheduled for a procedure on her throat (esophagus) to find out why she was having so much trouble eating and swallowing. However, they cancelled the procedure because her heart was racing at a very high rate (160-200 beats per minute). This was a very dangerous condition so they put her in Cardiac Critical Care to see if they could get the rate down. Drugs helped some, but they noticed that her lungs were also filling up quickly again.

Yesterday, they did a procedure to drain off another 1300cc of fluid from around the lungs and then inserted sterile talcum powder in the chest cavity to force the lung to adhere to the chest wall so new fluids could not form. In this way, the fluids would stop pressing on the lungs and heart. After the surgery, the heart rate dropped to about 125 beats per minute, but as of this morning, she was back up to 160+ and they are not sure why.

Dear friends, the reality (confirmed by her physicians) is that Susan is very near to the end of her journey. This morning she was sleeping heavily (drug induced) to maximize her comfort.

Her wish has always been that if and when the time came, it would not be drawn out. Please keep us in your prayers during the coming days. Pray for strength and ask that God would allow her to go home to Jesus quickly and with minimal discomfort if that is truly his will.

Susan sends her love (as do I) and I will be in contact again soon.

Blessings from our Lord Jesus Christ!

Gil

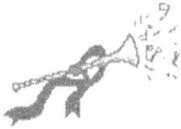

Sunday, January 14, 2007

Hello Everyone.

Susan's journey ended early this Sunday morning when she went home to be with her Lord Jesus Christ at 2:45 am.

She departed this earth quickly and peacefully, as was her wish and desire.

Although she never expected it because of all the cancer damage to her body, I was able to donate her corneas ... something she would have been absolutely thrilled about.

Thank you for being part of this journey with Susan. I pray that you have been touched and that the faith she shared has entered your heart and strengthened your own faith.

The details about the visitation and service are shown below. As part of our extended family, please join us if you can.

Blessings,

Gil

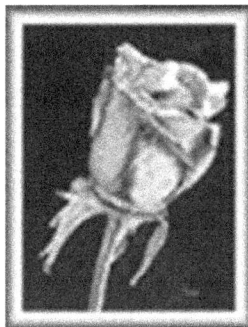

Susan's Song - Her Journey To Eternity

(Barbara) Susan Gerretsen, 46, wife of Gil Gerretsen, of North Barton Road, entered eternal life with her Lord and Savior Jesus Christ on Sunday, January 14, 2007 at St. Francis Hospital.

Born in Tampa, Florida, she was a devoted servant of her Lord. She used her four year battle with breast cancer as a chance to chronicle her journey and minister to many others through her writings.

Susan graduated from Hillsborough High School in Tampa and received her Bachelor of Nursing Degree from the University of South Carolina. She was a registered nurse with Bon Secours St. Francis where she worked as an operating room nurse.

Surviving in addition to her husband is her brother C. David Boggs of Houston, Texas.

The family will receive friends Friday, January 19 at John Knox Presbyterian Church in Greenville from 5:00 to 6:30pm. A celebration service honoring the life of Susan Gerretsen will follow at 7:00pm.